Breastfeeding for Beginners

The National
Childbirth
Trust
NCT

Breastfeeding for Beginners

Caroline Deacon

Thorsons

An Imprint of HarperCollins*Publishers*

in collaboration with National Childbirth Trust Publishing

Thorsons/National Childbirth Trust Publishing
Thorsons is an imprint of HarperCollins*Publishers*
77–85 Fulham Palace Road,
Hammersmith, London W6 8JB

The Thorsons website address is:
www.thorsons.com

and *Thorsons*
are trademarks of
HarperCollins*Publishers* Ltd

Published in collaboration with
National Childbirth Trust Publishing

10 9 8

© NCT Publishing 2002

Original photography by Anne Green-Armytage © 2002 NCT Publishing

Caroline Deacon asserts the moral right to be
identified as the author of this work

A catalogue record of this book is
available from the British Library

ISBN-13   978-0-00-713608-7
ISBN-10   0-00-713608-0

Printed and bound in Great Britain by
Martins the Printers Ltd, Berwick upon Tweed

Contents

Introduction

Why a book about breastfeeding?

What's there to learn about breastfeeding? In past times, women learnt by watching their mothers and sisters doing it. These days we don't always have our families at hand, and sometimes those who are nearby lack breastfeeding experience. Although breastfeeding is natural, it's not instinctive. Like riding a bike, learning can be difficult, even painful at first, if you get it wrong. Once you've mastered it, though, it's easy.

Choosing to breastfeed is not just a simple health issue. There are social and personal considerations too, and unfortunately our society is not always geared to supporting breastfeeding. Some health professionals are not able to help mothers adequately through the crucial early days, due to lack of time and training. Many women stop breastfeeding because their partners or other close family disapprove. It's important that your immediate family supports your decision to breastfeed; you are far more likely to get despondent if your partner waves a bottle under your nose whenever your baby cries. So get him to read this book too!

Some women do battle on against the odds, but no one should feel bad about not breastfeeding when they haven't had proper backup. If you are undecided about breastfeeding, or feel unsupported, talk to your health visitor or midwife, or phone a breastfeeding counsellor. We can listen and help you talk through your options; we'll support you in whatever decision you come to. A listening ear often helps.

This book has been written as a basic guide to breastfeeding your baby and you will find the emphasis is on practical information, rather than feelings and reflections. It's a pity we could not have included more of these in the book. I also feel sorry that pressure of space has meant no room for exploring the father's role in all this. Next time, perhaps!

Incidentally, throughout the book I have chosen to use the term 'weaning' to mean stopping breastfeeding as opposed to introducing solids, which is something that can happen alongside breastfeeding. I have also chosen to call the process of feeding your baby breastmilk substitutes 'formula feeding'. This is not a term I am entirely happy with, but the dried, processed cow's milk we feed to babies doesn't deserve the title 'breastmilk substitute', and although 'formula feeding' gives tinned milk more scientific credibility than I believe it deserves, it is, at present, the only term that mothers will readily recognize.

Caroline Deacon

NCT Breastfeeding Line 0870 444 8708

Ring this number for help with breastfeeding from a trained NCT counsellor, between 8am and 10pm, any day of the week, at only the cost of a national phone call.

Part 1

Getting Ready
for Breastfeeding

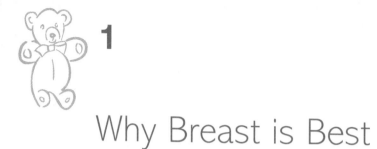

1

Why Breast is Best

You have probably heard that 'breast is best', but what does this saying actually mean?

It seems that nearly every day researchers make new discoveries about the benefits of breastfeeding. They've even found that people who were bottle-fed as babies are more likely to be snorers! This is not as daft as it sounds; apparently hard bottle teats can distort babies' mouths more than soft breast tissue, and this new shape can cause snoring, as well as giving some children crooked teeth.

While you're pregnant, your baby is totally dependent on your placenta for living, growing and developing. After the birth, your breasts take over where your womb left off, to continue giving him everything he needs to grow.

Breastmilk is a living fluid. It contains antibodies, hormones and many other substances we are only beginning to understand and which are impossible to store in tins. Your breastmilk changes continually, stimulating your baby's physical and intellectual development at critical times. At birth, for instance, your baby does not have a well-developed immune system. Instead, your body produces antibodies to fight specific germs with which your baby comes into contact, and passes these to him through your breastmilk. This is one reason why formula-fed babies are more likely to become ill.

No one has yet discovered the 'formula' for breastmilk, which is a complex, adaptable, living fluid with at least 300 different substances in it. The artificial babies' milk on sale in the supermarket is made from cow's milk, modified and then dried. When new substances are discovered in breastmilk, manufacturers may copy some artificially and add them to formula, but merely adding a substance is no guarantee that it works as it does in breastmilk. For instance, manufacturers add far more iron to formula milk than is found in breastmilk, but because this iron is in a form which is difficult to absorb, most of it is excreted. A lot needs to be added, therefore, if a baby is to receive enough iron.

The proteins found in cow's milk are not the same as those found in human milk, being ideal to help a calf grow rather than a human baby. Although formula manufacturers do alter cow's milk as far as possible to make it suitable for human babies, the proteins are still different, and can cause allergic reactions such as eczema and wheezing. Breastfed babies are far less likely to have respiratory tract infections or to wheeze. If you or your partner has any family history of allergy, asthma or eczema, then breastfeeding will help prevent your baby from developing the same conditions.

The carbohydrates in breastmilk pass through your baby's intestines faster, so there is less left in his gut to feed harmful bacteria. This may be one reason why tummy upsets are so common in formula-fed babies. It is also the reason your breastfed baby is much less likely to get constipated and why his stools smell sweeter. It may also be why some bottle-fed babies will go longer between feeds.

Your breastmilk's taste will change according to what you yourself are eating. If you have a curry, your milk will taste faintly of curry! Breastfed babies are thus acquiring the tastes they'll experience when they join their families at mealtimes later on.

We are only beginning to discover the long-term health benefits of breastfeeding. Studies have found, for instance, that these benefits continue long after breastfeeding stops. Intelligence tests of children aged seven or eight, who were premature and were given breastmilk, showed higher scores than those of other pre-term babies, although formula for pre-term babies has changed since then. IQ tests of full-term babies have also shown differences, but these are not always as clear-cut.

For you as well, breastfeeding brings benefits. If you breastfeed you are less likely to get pre-menopausal breast cancer, ovarian cancer or to suffer hip fractures when you are older. You are also more likely to get your figure back quickly!

If you are pregnant, your feelings about feeding may be hard to predict right now. You might feel you won't have enough energy after a long and difficult birth. Good support might not be available. However, if you are considering whether to breastfeed or not, or perhaps are having problems and are thinking about stopping, it can be motivating for you and those supporting you to know just some of the health benefits your baby will gain from being breastfed.

Research Findings about Breastfeeding

- Breastfed babies have a lower risk of respiratory infections, wheezing, urinary tract infections, glue ear, eczema, gastrointestinal infections, diarrhoea, prolonged colds and diabetes; they have better immune systems, a reduced risk of becoming allergic where there is a family history, and may have increased intelligence and better eyesight.
- Formula-fed babies are more likely to be hospitalized with respiratory or gastric problems.
- Mothers who breastfeed are less at risk of pre-menopausal breast cancer, ovarian cancer and hip fractures when older.
- Breastfeeding protects premature babies against the risk of death from neonatal necrotising enterocolitis.
- Breastfeeding may protect against cot death (sudden infant death syndrome, SIDS).
- There is also some evidence that children who were breastfed are less likely to have crooked teeth, inflammatory bowel disease and to develop cancer before the age of 15. The longer they were breastfed, the less likely they are to become diabetic.
- There is also some evidence that adults who were breastfed have less risk of coronary heart disease, multiple sclerosis, appendicitis and arthritis. They are more likely to experience a delay in any onset of coeliac disease.
- A Dundee study following up over 500 seven-year-olds found that the more breastmilk they received, the less likely they were ever to have had respiratory illnesses.

Your Questions Answered

Q I know that breastfeeding is supposed to be better for my baby, but I really can't face the idea of it. What can I do?

A Your baby does not have to take your breastmilk directly from your breasts to benefit. You could express your milk and give it to your baby in a cup or bottle, although this will be more time-consuming. Over several months, you might find it a challenge to keep your supply high enough to feed your baby with breastmilk alone. Perhaps you could keep an open mind until after your baby is born. Whatever your decision now, your breasts will still produce milk, so you might feel you would like to 'give it a go', even for just a few days.

Q I will need to give my baby formula on occasion; will this 'cancel out' the benefits of breastfeeding?

A Nearly all the research shows that the more breastmilk your baby gets, the more health benefits he will get. The other side of this means that babies who get breastmilk and formula are still benefiting from the breastmilk. The only exceptions are for diseases such as eczema and asthma, and for babies who are HIV-positive; research suggests that, for these illnesses, the longer you can avoid introducing anything other than breastmilk, the better. If you can wait until breastfeeding is established before introducing a bottle it will be easier – *see Chapter 13 on combined feeding.*

Q I didn't manage to breastfeed my baby, although I wanted to, and now I am worried about his future health...

A One thing to remember about research is that it shows trends. So, feeding your baby formula won't necessarily give him gastroenteritis, glue ear or any of these other problems; it just makes his chances of getting them higher. However, as a mother there are many other decisions you will have to make about your baby's future which may be a compromise – you may live near a busy road or have people who smoke around your child – all these will influence his health as well. Breastfeeding is one part of your baby's life; your love and care in many other ways are very important.

Because both my partner and I suffer from asthma, I was particularly keen to breastfeed. However, Thomas didn't gain weight well during the early weeks, and I was under a lot of pressure to top up with formula, which I didn't want to do. In the end, he started to gain and I did avoid the formula, and I think now that breastfeeding my babies has been one of the most satisfying experiences of my life.

Katherine, mother of Thomas, James and Megan

Myth or Fact?

You will Lose a Tooth for every Baby

Myth, nowadays, though it used to be true. Breastfeeding could deplete your calcium levels (especially with babies born close together) and on a poor diet this could lead to tooth loss, but this is rare now. Calcium levels in your bones increase again when you stop breastfeeding and your risk of osteoporosis may be lower if you have breastfed.

2

Breastfeeding and your Breasts

It can be reassuring to understand what happens to your breasts during pregnancy and breastfeeding.

It's nice to know that your baby will love your breasts no matter what size or shape they are. Nearly all breasts are capable of producing milk and have the same 'working' parts inside. It's easy to compare your breasts to those of 'Page Three' stars, and worry that yours are not all they should be. However, breasts in newspapers and magazines show only what our society currently thinks is 'ideal', instead of representing the huge range that is the reality for women.

Breasts contain 'lobes' which look a bit like bunches of grapes; these are where milk is made and stored. Each 'grape' has a tiny muscle running round it, which will squeeze milk out when needed. The lobes feed into ducts opening in the nipple. Every woman has between 15 and 25 of these, so that milk will come out of several tiny holes, a bit like water from a watering can.

The rest of the breast is made up of connective tissue, plus fat. Your breast size depends on the amount of fat, which is genetically determined and has no real function as far as breastfeeding is concerned. Therefore, size really doesn't matter for breastfeeding!

Nipples come in all shapes and sizes; most stick out, but flat or inverted nipples are also common. Surrounding your nipple is dark skin called the areola, which contains glands and hair follicles. Nearly all women have these hairs around their areolas, which may get darker or thicker during pregnancy. The Montgomery glands look like small bumps; these lubricate your nipple, so you don't need to prepare your breasts to feed, nor will you need to buy any special creams or lotions.

How your Breasts Change

The biggest changes to your breasts happen during pregnancy. Unless you were taking the contraceptive pill, you may already have been aware of some changes happening throughout your menstrual cycle, as your body prepared your breasts to feed a baby. For instance, your breasts may have become enlarged or sensitive just before your period. Once you started bleeding, these feelings subsided. After you conceive, these changes continue, and your body starts to produce the pregnancy hormone progesterone, which makes your breasts and areola swell. Your nipples may tingle and your breasts feel tender as your duct system starts to grow. The amount of change varies from woman to woman, and you may be quite unaware of any difference at first.

As your pregnancy progresses, the blood vessels under the surface of your breast skin become larger and more visible. These blue veins ensure your breasts will have enough blood supply to produce milk. The Montgomery glands also become more prominent, and you may even see secretions from them.

In late pregnancy, the levels of the hormone human placental lactogen (HPL) increase enormously as your body gets ready to produce milk. High levels of oestrogen will stop your body from producing large milk supplies while your pregnancy continues. However, from six months onwards, your body produces colostrum – the early milk, high in protein and antibodies, which your baby needs straight after birth.

Some women find tiny drops of colostrum dried on their nipples, forming a little crust, while other women can leak quite heavily. Although this might seem inconvenient, it's great to think that if your baby were born too soon, your body would be able to feed her. As birth approaches, your nipples and areola become far darker and more obvious, almost like a target for your baby to aim at!

New mothers are faced with a dazzling array of creams, sprays and lotions, all of which imply that breastfeeding is going to hurt and that it needs lots of medications to keep going. In fact, it is not normal for breastfeeding to hurt, and you do not need to buy any special creams or lotions. Your nipple skin may even react to some of these, so if you want to use a cream or lotion, test it in the crook of your arm first to see if you get any adverse reaction.

Looking after your Breasts

Breasts have no muscles, and the ligaments that support your breast tissue can easily become stretched. Once this happens, your breasts will sag and nothing can lift them up again. So if having firm, upright breasts is important to you, you will need to invest in a good supporting bra, ideally from the moment you realize you're expecting, as pregnancy will make your breasts heavier. Avoid under-wired bras, as these can damage your growing ducts.

Your Guide to Buying a Bra that Fits Well

Many women underestimate their cup size, but a cup that's too small won't offer adequate support. If you're used to under-wired bras, it is

hard for an unwired one to feel anything like as supportive. A professional fitting can help.

- Bras have two measurements – cup size (A indicates small cup, H large), and ribcage or chest size (32 small, 40 large). If your breasts are large you will need a bigger *letter*, but if your body is large, you will probably need a bigger *number*. As a general rule, the cup size also increases as the chest size increases. Thus a 36B will often have the same cup size as a 34C or a 38A, the difference being how loose the bra feels across the back.
- If you're measuring yourself, take one line around your ribcage, just under your breasts. This is your chest size. Next measure round your breasts loosely while wearing a bra. The difference between this and your ribcage will give you your cup size. Roughly speaking, five inches means an A cup, and every extra inch increases the cup. Thus an eight-inch difference means a D cup.
- If the cup feels baggy and it seems you are not filling it properly, undo the bra again, lean forward and drop your breasts down into the cups. Then do it up again – this often takes up the slack.
- Your bra strap at the back should be low and level, not riding up, and normally the straps supporting the cups should be tightened slightly, so they are neither fully up nor down. They should be wide enough not to dig into your shoulders.
- A bra for pregnancy should give firm support, and allow for expansion, so it should initially fit on the tightest adjustment across the back.
- Extension straps, which clip onto your bra's own hooks and eyes, can tide you over the last few weeks of pregnancy.
- Your bra might cut in under your breasts as your bump gets higher and higher. Try fastening the bottom hook on a slacker setting than the others, or leave that hook undone altogether. Once the baby's head engages, it should get more comfortable.

If you are exercising during and after pregnancy, your breasts shouldn't 'jig up and down'. Tighten the straps, and watch yourself in a mirror. Try to choose exercises that avoid straining your breast ligaments – cycling is probably better than jogging, for example.

Buying a bra for breastfeeding

Wearing a badly fitting bra while breastfeeding can cause blocked ducts, mastitis and even abscesses, so getting the right size is important. There's no need to buy a nursing or feeding bra, but you should be able to free your breast totally when feeding, which for a normal bra means taking it off – not always convenient! Feeding bras have special zip or drop-cup fastenings that allow you to undo one cup at a time, without undoing the bra.

- Don't buy a feeding bra any earlier than six weeks before your baby is due.
- If you get fitted while pregnant, your feeding bra should only just do up on the last hook, otherwise it will be too slack after the birth.
- Bear in mind you will probably want to be able to undo it and do it up again discreetly, preferably with one hand while balancing your baby on your knee! During the fitting you could try undoing and redoing the different styles under a T-shirt, to give you an idea.

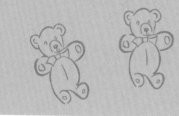

Your Questions Answered

Q Will I definitely need a new bra, and if so, how soon?

A You may well need a new bra as soon as you are pregnant. An average woman will gain about two cup sizes, and expand across the chest at least two inches during the nine months of pregnancy.

Q Which feeding bra is better – zip or drop-cup opening?

A Zip fastening is often better than a drop-cup opening if you have large breasts. Protect your breast when doing it up by putting your thumb between you and the zip. Some women are put off by zip opening bras because they are so obviously for feeding. If you prefer a drop-cup bra, make sure all the cup comes away and that the retaining strap is very loose, so it won't cut into your breast while feeding.

I've always had small breasts, but pregnancy and breastfeeding changed them from an A cup to a double D, which I loved! After Eleanor was born, my figure was the best it's ever been.

Sarah, mother of Eleanor, Jack and Charlotte

Myth or Fact?

Breastfeeding makes your Breasts Sag

Myth. The change happens during pregnancy. Minimize sagging by investing in some good bras.

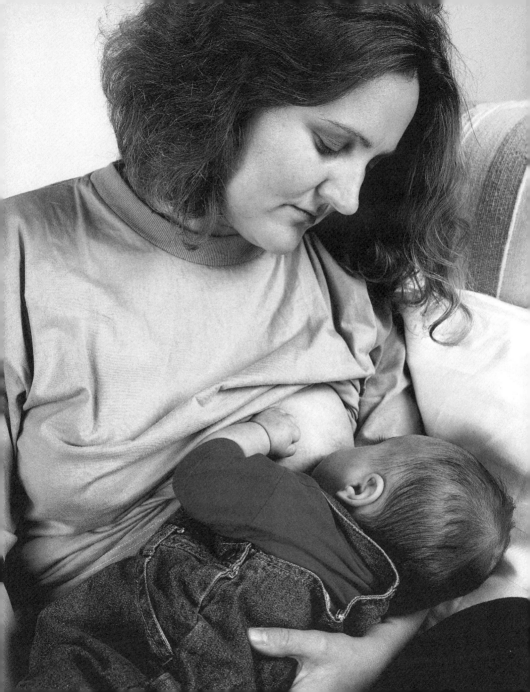

Part 2

Understanding Breastfeeding

3

How Breastfeeding Works

How your body produces milk to feed your baby.

While you're breastfeeding, your body produces two hormones, oxytocin and prolactin.

Prolactin ensures that your body creates more milk to replace what your baby has just taken, so you'll never run out. Prolactin levels are often higher at night and make you feel sleepy, so when you get up to feed your baby, your body makes sure you can get back to sleep easily.

When your body thinks that your baby needs to feed, oxytocin will make the muscles around your ducts contract (*see Chapter* 2), pushing milk down from deep in your breast to where your baby can get it. This is called the 'let down reflex', which you may be able to feel as a tingling sensation; it might even be strong enough to feel painful. Some women are completely unaware of their let down reflex, but all women will let down milk. Even a baby who is not well positioned at the breast may get a reasonable amount of milk purely from what his mother lets down (although in the long run he will not get enough milk).

Once breastfeeding is established, your let down can be triggered even when your baby is not with you – perhaps by hearing another baby cry, or by thinking about your own baby. Your milk may gush or spurt out, so you might need to wear breast pads when you are out and about, or have a cloth ready for mopping up from your other breast when you are feeding your baby.

Oxytocin also helps your womb contract during the days after the birth, so it can return to its pre-pregnancy size. Some women find these contractions painful – hence the term 'afterpains', especially for second or subsequent babies. If you find these strong, ask your midwife for some painkillers; the pain will only last for a few days.

Oxytocin is also the hormone that makes you feel good when making love. Even when you are not pregnant or breastfeeding, your breasts are connected through your autonomic nervous system to your womb and clitoris, which is why some women can reach orgasm through nipple stimulation alone. When you make love, milk may spurt or run from your breasts as your oxytocin levels increase. If this is a problem, it can help to feed your baby before you make love.

What is Breastmilk?

From about 20 weeks of pregnancy until several days after your baby's birth, your breasts produce a straw-coloured milk called colostrum. Although the quantities you will produce are tiny – usually no more than a teaspoon per feed – it will give your baby a real boost as he enters the world because it's rich in antibodies. It also acts as a laxative to help your baby pass meconium – his first, black and sticky, stools. Feeding your baby often in those early days will also help him avoid jaundice, because colostrum helps your baby expel bilirubin (the orangey pigment) from his bowels.

After a few days of feeding, your colostrum will be replaced by mature breastmilk; this is often referred to as your milk 'coming in'. From now on, at every feed, each breast will start with fore milk (the milk which comes in *before*), which is dilute and thirst-quenching, gradually thickening into hind milk (the milk which follows *behind*), which is packed with calories. So when your baby latches on, first he has a refreshing drink, then he gets down to a satisfying meal of hind milk, which helps him grow at an enormous rate. Therefore, if you limit your baby's time at the breast, or swap sides too soon, he won't get as much of the hind milk as he needs to grow, and will be hungry again very quickly.

Human breastmilk – whether colostrum or mature breastmilk – will not look like the milk you buy to drink – not surprising, as a baby calf is quite a different prospect from a 7lb human baby! Some women worry that their milk looks too thin because they expect it to look like cow's milk, but be assured that your milk is perfect for your baby.

Not only does your milk change during each feed, it also varies with circumstances. If your baby is breastfed, you are able to continuously monitor harmful organisms in his environment by pouring specific antibodies into your breastmilk. In other words, breastmilk carries antibodies to combat whichever germs you come into contact with that day. Your baby's immune system is immature during his first year and he cannot fight infections as well as you can, so you pass your own selected antibodies to your baby through your breastmilk.

Of course, unwanted substances may pass through your breastmilk too. So just as you did in pregnancy, you should consider carefully what you are eating and drinking, avoiding any unnecessary medication (*see Chapter 7, 'Breastfeeding and your diet'*).

As your breasts prepare to step up supply, changing from low-volume colostrum to higher-volume mature breastmilk, they become engorged with blood, and you may feel uncomfortable, hot, and find it difficult to latch your baby on as well as before. Often the accompanying changes in hormone levels will make you feel weepy – this is known as the 'baby blues'. It will pass within 24 to 48 hours, never to return, but in the meantime, feeding your baby as often as possible helps it pass (*see Chapter* 10 *for more on engorgement*).

How do I Make Enough Breastmilk?

It's quite simple to make enough milk: let your baby decide when he needs to eat, and when he has had enough. Only he is capable of deciding how much he really needs. The more you feed, the higher your prolactin levels and therefore the more milk you will produce – you can't run out. 'Saving it up' for later will actually mean you will have less than you need. This system of producing more milk whenever your baby feeds is often called 'supply and demand' or baby-led feeding.

In the early days, when your body is trying to work out how much milk your baby is going to ask for, avoid giving your baby other fluids as this will mean he has less room for milk. Jaundice, for instance, is best treated with breastmilk, rather than water or formula milk.

Your Questions Answered

Q Does feeding my baby on demand mean I am spoiling him?

A If you think of it as baby-led feeding rather than demand feeding, it sounds better! If you think about it, you too work on 'supply and demand'. When you are short of supplies, your tummy 'demands' more – it tells you that you are hungry. When your baby is hungry, he will let you know ('demands'). Your breasts then get to know how much your baby needs and when, and will 'supply' the amount of milk he needs. Your baby will be happier if he is fed when he's hungry and not kept waiting.

Q So is it always my baby who decides when to feed?

A No – you and your baby will form a two-way feeding partnership. If your breasts feel full, then you need to feed, so you can 'demand' that your baby feeds and he will usually oblige. If you skip a feed, or go too long between feeds, you may get engorged, so feed your baby when you need to relieve this feeling of being over full. You don't need to wait until he asks every time.

> I have always thought breastfeeding is very convenient – hot milk on tap at the right moment! Amanda was a very slow feeder at the beginning, so breastfeeding used to take a long time, but she did improve. The other two were fine from the start. That is the thing – it does always get much better and easier as time goes on.

Abigail, mother to Amanda, Ben and Katie

Myth or Fact?

If your Baby Feeds for too Long he will use up your Milk

Myth. Your baby cannot use up your milk. More is produced as soon as it is removed. But if you need to cut feeds short occasionally, you can do. Remember, breastfeeding is a two-way relationship.

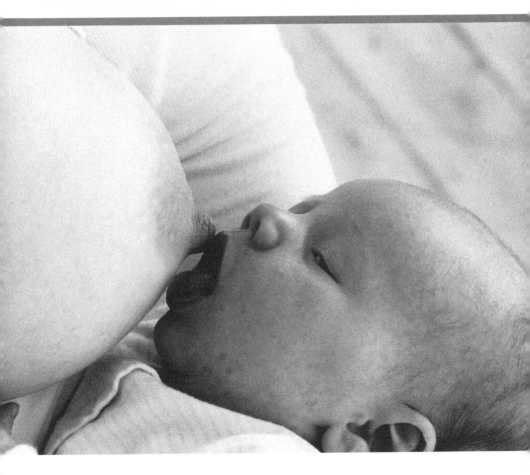

4

Positioning your Baby at your Breast

Although breastfeeding is natural, good positioning and attachment is something both you and your baby need to learn. If you have an idea of what you're aiming for, it really does help.

Have you ever wondered why it's called 'breastfeeding', not 'nipple feeding'? Because your baby feeds from a mouth full of breast – she doesn't suck on your nipples. In fact, she needs a mouthful large enough for your nipple to come into contact with her soft palate, which is at the back of the roof of her mouth. When your baby's soft palate is stimulated, she instinctively starts to move her jaws so that she can breastfeed. If your nipple is not far enough in, it makes contact instead with your baby's hard palate (peek in her mouth and you will see ridges). Your nipple would soon get sore pressed into that part of your baby's mouth.

- Your baby is born with a rooting reflex, which means that she will search for your breast, mouth gaping just as it needs to be to latch on properly.
- The other instinct at work is to suck automatically when her soft palate is stimulated.

Before you begin, get comfortable. You could be sitting in the same position for quite a while! It's easier in the beginning to sit upright, so choose a chair which will support you; slouching back tends to pull your breast out of baby's mouth. You might need cushions or pillows to help you get upright.

Your feet should reach the floor so that your knees are level or even slightly raised to give your baby a nice cosy lap. A small stool or some telephone directories under your feet may help.

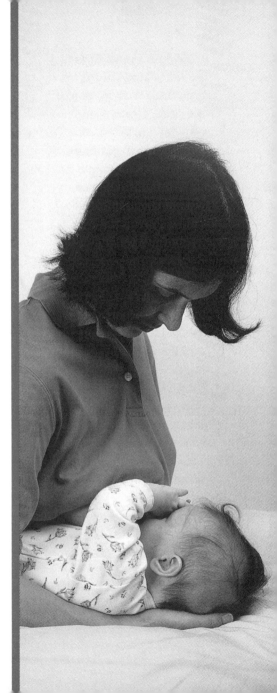

If your breasts are high then you might find a pillow, or even two, useful to rest your arms on when bringing your baby level with your breasts. It may be easier to get your baby latched on first, and then tuck the pillows under your arms, otherwise the pillows can get between the two of you when you are trying to get started.

The most common position for holding a baby is across your tummy, but you could hold her 'underarm', especially if she's small, or if you've had a caesarean section and need to protect your tummy. You will need to have several cushions between you and the chair back if feeding underarm, so your baby can stretch out without pushing herself off your breast. If she's across your tummy, you can support her head on your forearm (not the crook of your arm).

Next time you have a drink in your hand, put your chin as near to your chest as you can. Now try swallowing. Impossible, isn't it? But a baby who is too far round, who latches on with your nipple facing her lower lip, has to try to swallow like this. Now try swallowing your drink with your head back, so your throat is open. Much easier. Try to remember this when feeding your baby – she can't adjust her position so her throat is open, but you can do it for her.

To help your baby latch on well, turn her so that she is facing you, 'tummy to tummy'. Hold her so her back is straight, her bottom tucked in and her nose level with your nipple. Wait until her mouth gapes, then move her quickly onto your breast. Once she is on, her gape should still be wide. There should be more of your breast in her mouth below your nipple than above it (ask someone to look). Her bottom lip will be curled back and her chin will dig into your breast, but her nose will be relatively clear. You may see her jaw chomping steadily and powerfully – maybe even making her ears wiggle up and down. If her cheeks are hollowing then she hasn't got a good mouthful. If she's feeding well, she'll be relaxed and calm, and if you gently peep in the corner of her mouth you will see that her tongue is covering her lower gums.

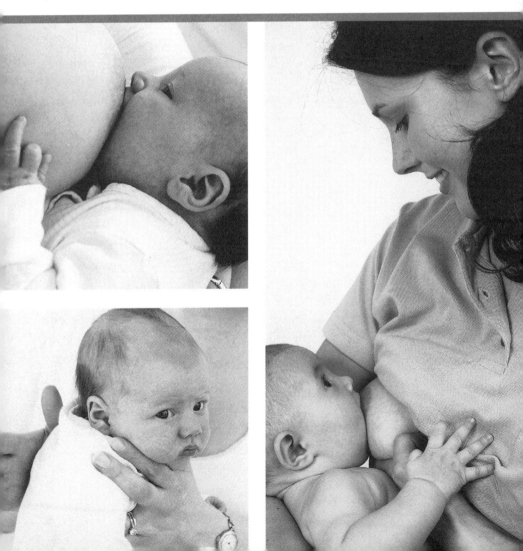

Breastfed babies don't aways need winding, but if you think she needs to burp sit her up and, supporting her chest and chin, gently rub her back (*see also Chapter 9, Crying, Colic and your Breastfeeding Baby*).

It can be restful to feed your baby lying down, but this can be difficult to do at first without help. Lie on your side, supporting your head, shoulders and lower arm with pillows. Once you're ready, get someone to place your baby close to you, 'tummy to tummy', so her nose is level with your nipple. Now you can, with your upper arm, cuddle her bottom in close. Once she roots for the breast – her mouth gapes wide – draw her in closer with your hand on her upper back, and her mouth should contact your breast.

Passing the Time

You can be sure that the minute you settle down to feed your baby, the phone will ring! Many women don't realize how long they will spend actually sitting feeding the baby in those early weeks – just when all your friends want to ring and chat about the birth. After you get proficient at breastfeeding you will eventually manage to feed with one hand free, and then you can spend time catching up with your mates on the phone. You can also catch up on all those films you've recorded but not got around to watching – have one ready loaded in the machine with the remote controls next to your feeding chair. (You may also find you are thirsty while feeding your baby, so it's a good idea to have a drink of water to hand.)

Top Tips for Correct Positioning and Attachment

- *Support your baby* **spine in line.** Hold her so that her back and shoulders are straight. Avoid holding the back of her head, which would push her chin towards her chest, making it difficult for her to open her mouth wide. Also, most babies don't like having their heads held.
- *Hold your baby so you are both* **tummy to tummy.** She will not be able to feed well if she has to turn her head sideways.
- *Align your baby's head so she's* **nose to nipple.** Don't hold her mouth to nipple, as would seem logical, because once she is on your breast, her chin would be pushed towards her chest and her throat would close, making swallowing difficult and slow. Your nipple needs to contact the roof of her mouth to make her feed properly, and needs to be far enough back to avoid contact with her hard palate – that bony ridge at the front of her mouth – which would rub against and hurt your nipple.
- **Wait for the gape.** Wait until her mouth is really wide open – imagine she is about to bite on an apple – and then draw her swiftly onto your breast.
- **Chin in.** Her chin will contact your breast first, digging well in, and leaving her nose clear.

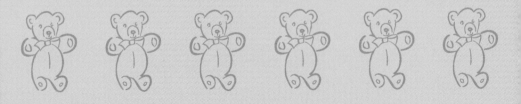

Your Questions Answered

 Q Why does my baby feed for so long? She can stay on for hours, but she is not gaining weight very well.

A This could be due to positioning which is not quite right. If your baby has to turn her head sideways, or has her chin on her chest, swallowing will take a long time. Check that her throat can be open, and her neck extended, so she can swallow quickly and easily.

 Q Can my baby breathe OK when she is feeding?

A Babies have tiny noses with flared nostrils – ideal for breastfeed-ing. If your baby can't breathe, she will let you know by coming off your breast. If she does this, then consider positioning and attachment: is her chin against your breast, is her bottom tucked in close to your body? If her body is too far away from you it can make her nose sink into your breast. If she's finding it hard to breathe because she has a snuffle, then ask your GP for some nose drops, which you can give her just before a feed.

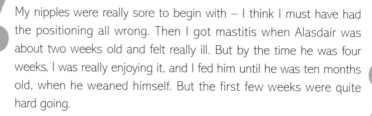

My nipples were really sore to begin with – I think I must have had the positioning all wrong. Then I got mastitis when Alasdair was about two weeks old and felt really ill. But by the time he was four weeks, I was really enjoying it, and I fed him until he was ten months old, when he weaned himself. But the first few weeks were quite hard going.

Caroline, mother of Alasdair

Myth or Fact?

If your Baby Feeds for too Long, She will give you sore Nipples

Myth. If positioning is fine, then you and your baby can feed for as long as you both want to, without soreness. Sore nipples can happen for other reasons, but not length of feed.

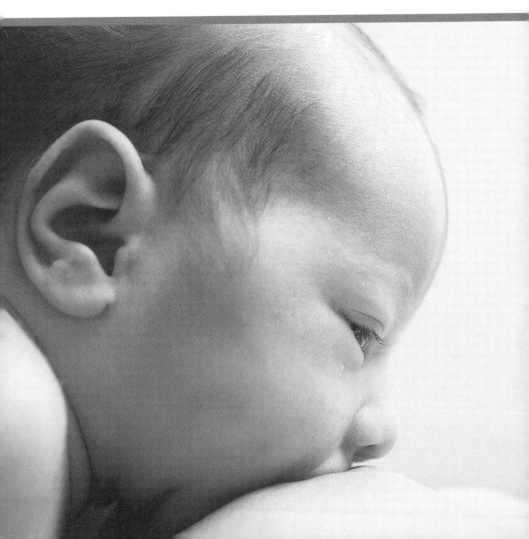

5

Getting Off to a Good Start

Often, all it takes is one really good feed, and you and your baby will soon become 'experts'.

If you can put your baby to your breast soon after the birth, it will help both of you get off to a good start. Research indicates that when newborn babies are cuddled close to the breast with their skin touching their mother's skin, starting breastfeeding is easier. You might want to request this early skin-to-skin contact on your birth plan so that hospital staff don't whisk your baby away for routine tasks during this crucial time.

Once your baby has been born, hold him close to your breast and see if he 'roots' – looks for your breast with his mouth open wide. His suckling instinct will be strong, so he could latch on well during this cuddling time. If he's not in the mood, then simply holding him skin-to-skin will start to stimulate your milk supply, as well as giving you both a chance to get to know each other. After all, he may prefer to look around at this world he's entered before he's ready to feed.

After these early moments, your baby may well sleep for long periods on his first day. Not surprising, really, as birth is also tiring for him. Although you may feel worn out, you will also be feeling 'high' and probably unable to sleep. Your baby may not seem interested in food at first, but you can spend as much time as you feel you want to in skin-to-skin contact, offering him the breast during his brief moments of alertness.

The Effects of Labour

- If you were given pethidine during labour, especially only a few hours before the birth, it can reduce your baby's suckling reflex for several days. This can mean breastfeeding will take longer to get established, so in the meantime, have skin-to-skin contact as much as you can.
- A caesarean section shouldn't affect your baby's ability to breastfeed, but it may make it harder for you to hold him in a good position. Many women find an underarm hold works well, and lying on your side can also be comfortable. Do ask for help to get into a comfortable position.
- An assisted delivery – forceps or ventouse – can give your baby a headache, and being held in certain positions or even suckling could be painful for him. He will need you to be patient, perhaps experimenting with different positions.

Early Days

At first, your baby will feed little and often. His tiny tummy, which is only the size of a walnut, can't hold much. Also he is learning how to feed and tires quickly, so feeding will occupy much of your time until he gets the hang of it.

Some babies are quite sleepy after the birth. Your midwife may suggest waking your baby to feed him, as sleepy babies can get lethargic and 'forget' to feed. You may particularly need to wake a small baby, or one who has had pethidine, to make sure he is getting enough to eat.

Jaundice is common in newborn babies, when they look as if they have a lovely suntan. Breastfeeding as often as possible helps this pass, but again you may need to wake him to feed as jaundice does

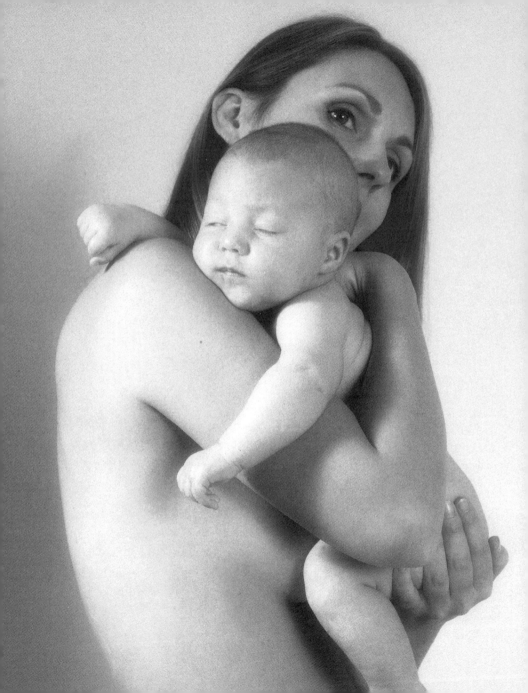

make babies sleepy. Your midwife will be able to tell whether the jaundice is mild, or severe enough to need treatment.

Swaddling

If your baby thrashes about when you are trying to get him latched on, you could try swaddling him to keep his arms from getting in the way. Lay him on his back on a thin blanket with the edge across his shoulders. Bring the two top corners down to tuck tightly under his bottom. This will pin his arms by his sides. If he enjoys being swaddled, you can wrap him in another blanket for extra warmth and comfort after the feed has finished.

Going Home

If your baby was born in hospital, the idea of taking him to his new home is exciting but daunting. In fact, it can often feel easier to breastfeed at home where you're comfortable and relaxed. Both of you will be tired after the birth and need to rest, so you will need someone there to give you lots of practical help and positive encouragement. Make sure you get the help you need.

Getting through the Early Days

There's no doubt that breastmilk gives your baby the best possible start in life, and new mothers can find this thought keeps them going if they are finding breastfeeding difficult. Perhaps you might like to have some books or leaflets to read about the benefits of breastfeeding in your hospital bag. Remind yourself why you want to breastfeed; tell yourself how much easier breastfeeding is going to be in the long run, as well as all the benefits you are giving your baby.

The problem is that there has been so much bottle-feeding in the last few generations that some health professionals lack the confidence and skills needed to help women breastfeed successfully. Some women who stop breastfeeding early, or who never managed to get started, later feel regret and guilt, but it wasn't their fault – the system failed them. If you find you are having problems and your health professional isn't helping effectively, do look around for other sources of help. Consult a different midwife, or contact a breastfeeding counsellor. The National Childbirth Trust has also set up a national telephone line that you can call any day between 8am and 10pm for help with breastfeeding: 0870 444 8708.

Many hospitals now make a real effort to support breastfeeding, and some have adopted the 'Ten Steps to Successful Breastfeeding' – a charter drawn up by the World Health Organization. These hospitals can be awarded 'Baby Friendly Status', which means they have practices in place to support breastfeeding (*see Appendix 3 for the Ten Steps*). If your hospital is not 'baby friendly' then you might want to incorporate the ten steps in your birth plan.

Research also shows that you are far more likely to continue to breastfeed if the people close to you support your decision. Talk through issues with your partner. You might like to think together about various questions: how will you handle night feeds in the early days? Where is your baby going to sleep? When you are out and about as a family, how will you both feel about you breastfeeding in public? Remember, it is perfectly possible, once you have had some practice, to feed your baby discreetly.

It is not just your partner who has an opinion about breastfeeding – your baby's grandparents can feel positive or negative as well. Your mother may feel ambivalent if her own breastfeeding experiences were unhappy or if she was persuaded to bottle-feed. If you can, have a good chat about it all before the baby arrives; it can clear the air and she will be more able to support you fully when you need it.

As soon as your baby is born, you are likely to have lots of visitors. This is understandable, but many mothers have said how difficult they found breastfeeding while dealing with dozens of visitors. In the early days, you and your baby may be all fingers and thumbs when breastfeeding, and it can be hard to feed discreetly in front of other people. For the first couple of weeks, you will also feel tired and in need of rest. If you are rushing about making tea and coffee, or trying to tidy up, you will not be giving your milk supply the best chance of getting established. Perhaps you might want to restrict the number of visitors until you feel comfortable about feeding in front of other people.

Once you are out of hospital, it can be useful to meet up with other mums who are breastfeeding, for support. Perhaps the women you meet at antenatal classes would like to keep in touch, or you could exchange phone numbers with women you meet in hospital. The NCT runs a national network of postnatal support groups, putting new mums in touch with each other for regular support and socializing. You'll find more information at the back of this book. Ask your health visitor for details of your local mother and baby groups, or for any local breastfeeding drop-in centres.

Your Questions Answered

Q I've heard my local hospital tests all babies for hypoglycaemia. Is this good?

A Unless your baby is ill, premature or small for dates, or unless you are diabetic, then your baby is unlikely to develop hypogly-caemia (low blood sugar), and routine blood sugar testing is usu-ally unhelpful. If there are worries about your baby being hypoglycaemic, perhaps because he's sleeping too much and not feeding, then clinical observation and examination by a paedia-trician is usually a better option. Your breastmilk is likely to be the best nourishment for him, so if he is not feeding well, you can express some milk which can be given from a cup or syringe.

Q How can I tell if sore nipples are just normal, or if we've got the positioning wrong?

A During the first few days of breastfeeding, you may feel some dis-comfort. Some women find the strong sensation as the baby latches on a bit of a shock. For other women, their nipple skin is extra sensi-tive for about a week after the birth, and this can make breastfeed-ing feel uncomfortable. However, the baby should not damage or distort your nipple in any way. When he finishes a feed, if your nipple looks squashed, blanched or with a ridge pattern on it, then he has not got enough of your breast in his mouth. A good rule of thumb is to wait for 30 seconds after your baby has latched on, and if it still hurts, then take him off and try again. (Break the suction first by putting your little finger in the corner of his mouth.) Make sure you get lots of help from a midwife or breastfeeding counsellor.

Q How long does it take to get used to breastfeeding?

A This varies from one mother to another. Some mothers feel at ease with breastfeeding in a few days but others take several weeks to feel they've become skilful.

I don't think my caesars made breastfeeding any different. In fact, I think I had considerably fewer problems than many of my friends. I used a beanbag to prop them up and that protected my scar. With Georgina, my first baby, I had cracked nipples, but that was more to do with lacking any idea of how to go about breastfeeding than to do with the caesar.

Kerry, mother of Georgina, Charlie and Hamish, all born by emergency caesarean section

Myth or Fact?

Many Women find Breastfeeding painful for the First Week

Fact. It seems many women's nipples are extra sensitive for a few days after birth. However, poor latching on (or attachment) is the most frequent cause of sore nipples, so it's always worth asking a breastfeeding counsellor to check.

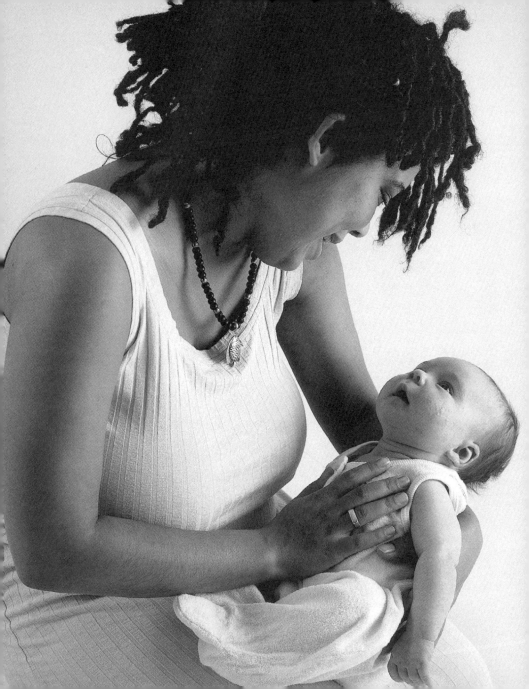

Part 3

Breastfeeding in your Life

6

How Much and How Often?

A common worry many new mothers have is how often their babies need breastfeeding.

Long ago, babies were carried around all the time and fed whenever they seemed hungry. Over the past 100 years or so, various breastfeeding regimes have come and gone, so now many mothers feel completely confused about what babies want or need. A generation ago, mothers were told to feed babies for 20 minutes only, every four hours. The advice was well meant; the 'expert' in this case hoped to make being a mother easier by imposing routines on baby from day one. For a few it worked, but other babies couldn't get enough milk and were very unhappy.

This idea – feeding for 20 minutes every four hours – came from observing calves, but babies' needs are different from those of cows. For instance, a newborn's tummy is only the size of a walnut, so it empties quite quickly. Also, breastmilk is easily and quickly digested. Unlike calves, human babies are helpless and expect to be carried around near their mothers' breasts, feeding more or less continuously while their mothers get on with their lives.

Baby-led Feeding

Research shows that your body will make the right amount of milk for your baby, if you let her feed when she asks. If you try to impose a feeding pattern that suits you, your body will produce the amount of milk you let it, which may not be the same. Only your baby knows how hungry she is, and how much breastmilk she needs for her hunger to be satisfied.

If you think about it, this is how you feed too. Your body tells you when you are hungry, when you are thirsty, and when you are full up. You can go to the fridge and help yourself; your baby has to signal to you to put her to your breast, and she will usually come off when she has had enough.

If you have worries about how long your baby takes over her feeds, it can help to think about the adult she will grow up to be. Sometimes adults like us have a quick snack, or just a little drink. Other times we are really hungry and will enjoy a big scoff. Occasionally we go out to a restaurant and sit for a few hours, enjoying a meal with friends. How would you feel if the waiter rushed up and said, 'Right you've had 20 minutes, you must have finished now'?

That isn't to say that if baby wants her own version of a three-course feast when you are about to go out, you always have to agree. If it is not convenient at that point, and you are happy to tell your baby to wait a few minutes, or to have a shorter feed, that's fine, as long as you also agree to sit down for a long meal and sociable cuddle at another time.

Comfort Feeding

Some mothers worry that their baby is 'just comfort feeding'. They wonder how they can tell when she's breastfeeding because she's hungry, and when she's feeding for other reasons. Again, think about yourself. How many of those chocolate biscuits or cups of coffee do you have because you are hungry or thirsty, and how many do you have for 'comfort'? Do you only eat and drink at mealtimes and because you really need to, or do you sometimes have meals or snacks to be sociable, or to relieve boredom?

For a baby, breastfeeding is not just about nutrition; it is also about warmth and closeness and learning to be a social human being. Researchers notice that breastfeeding babies interact with their mothers, pausing while she talks, replying by sucking. They believe that feeding a baby teaches the give and take of communication and forms the basis of learning human speech.

Try not to feel pressured into feeding your baby according to someone else's idea of the right pattern. If you feel happy with the way breastfeeding is going, and if your baby is healthy and growing, then you are doing it right. Remember, you can't spoil a baby (what she wants is what she needs), or overfeed a breastfed baby. If you feel unhappy with feeding (perhaps, for example, you don't like feeding her as much as it seems she wants), then talk it through with a breastfeeding counsellor. She won't tell you what you must do, but she'll help you explore your options so that you can feel right in doing what you want to do.

Is my Baby Getting Enough to Eat?

Wouldn't it be great if breasts had indicators on them, like plastic bottles, so we could see just how much milk a baby gets at each feed! But your body fed your baby for nine months inside your womb without you thinking about it. It wouldn't make sense if your body couldn't continue to provide all her nutritional needs afterwards. If you're worried, think:

- Does your baby seem healthy and alert?
- Does she have six to eight wet reusable nappies a day, or four to six disposable ones?
- Is her poo bright yellow, sweet smelling and the consistency of scrambled eggs?

These are all signs that your baby is doing well. Most babies, unless they are very small, premature, jaundiced or otherwise unwell, will let you know in no uncertain terms if they are not getting enough milk.

Baby's Weight Gain

If your baby doesn't seem to gain weight the same way as the charts:

- Look at her overall pattern. If she lost more than 10 per cent of her birth weight in the beginning, for instance, it will take her longer to catch up. If she put on a lot of weight for a couple of weeks, then it may well slow down a bit in the following weeks.
- Sometimes your baby's weight appears to fluctuate because the health visitor has used different scales, or weighed her with or without clothes or nappy.
- Think about her bowels – if she did a big poo just before weighing, that would affect her weight.
- It is important to look at growth in length and head circumference over a period of months too, since these can be more accurate and positive signs of normal development than just focusing on weight, which is about body fat.

Not Enough Milk?

Many mothers worry whether they have enough milk. It is worth remembering that even women who are starving or severely malnourished manage to feed their babies purely on breastmilk. Your body can nearly always produce enough milk for your baby, if you allow her to breastfeed as often as she asks.

If you need to increase your supply, then try cutting down on everything you are doing over a 48-hour period. Rest as much as you can, feed your baby as often as possible, and eat plenty of nutritious meals and snacks. If your milk supply was low, it should increase to the right amount after this intensive period.

When Feeding Suddenly Increases

If your baby has always seemed content, but then suddenly appears to want to feed all the time, there are several possible reasons:

- She will have 'appetite spurts' at certain stages of her development. Common times seem to be around two weeks, six weeks and twelve weeks, although it will vary from baby to baby. At these times, she will want to increase your milk supply to carry her through the next few weeks. Try the suggestion above for increasing your milk supply.
- When your baby is ill or teething, she may want to feed a lot. She may feed for what seems like all the time for a day or so before she develops an illness. Again, try to be led by your baby; when she is ill, breastmilk is the best thing for her.

Your Questions Answered

Q My baby seems to take a long time to feed — sometimes I am sitting feeding her for over an hour! Is this normal? I wonder if I don't have enough milk.

A If you didn't have enough milk, your baby would be upset — she wouldn't be content at the breast. In the first couple of weeks, while you and your baby are learning, then you could expect some long feeds. Also, if your baby is quite small, or has been ill, then it will take her longer. However, feeding often takes a long time when the baby is not positioned well. It can look as if she has a good mouthful of breast, and is feeding happily, but if you are holding her so that it is difficult for her to swallow, this will slow things up. With a small or very young baby, positioning is far more crucial than with an older baby. Ask your midwife or breast-feeding counsellor to have a look at how your baby is feeding.

Q How do I get my baby into a regular feeding routine?

A If you need to get your baby into a regular feeding pattern, it is best to wait until she is a well-established breastfeeder before you try to extend the spaces between feeds gradually, and per-haps also to keep her awake for longer during a feed so that she will take more. It may help to look on the new pattern as one that you and your baby negotiate together, rather than one you impose on her.

Jack used to want to feed for hours in the evenings. Because he was my second, I knew I should just go with it and wait for that need to pass. So I watched a lot of telly and he grew out of it soon enough.

Sarah

Myth or Fact?

Babies should be able to Feed for 10 Minutes on each Side, every Three Hours

Myth. Only a few babies will be happy with this regime, and trying to regulate feeds to fit this pattern is likely to create problems. Most babies have varying intervals between feeds; sometimes several feeds are clustered together. Some babies feed fast while others feed more slowly.

7

Breastfeeding and your Diet

Looking after yourself is important when you have a baby, so here are some suggestions about what to eat and drink when breastfeeding.

Everyone has their own theory about how many extra calories you need to make milk, but we doubt whether you will have time to count them in those early weeks! The fact is that it normally works well if you eat and drink to appetite. Your body will tell you what it needs.

Unless you are severely malnourished, your body will produce nutritious milk containing everything needed to feed your growing baby. If your diet is deficient in anything, your own health will suffer before your baby's. Generally speaking, a healthy daily diet would have wholegrain foods, like wholemeal bread and pasta or brown rice, as the main part of your meal, with a good variety of fresh fruit and vegetables and some protein. It's good practice to avoid too many fatty, sugary or refined foods.

Unfortunately, making yourself something decent to eat is often the first task that gets neglected when you are trying to adapt to life with a new baby, but you will quickly get exhausted if you skip meals. If you wait until your body reminds you that you haven't eaten for a while, you may already have become depleted. Try to pick up on the early signs of hunger, or perhaps you could set an alarm to remind you to eat or drink every two or three hours. This pattern should keep your blood sugar constant, which has the added bonus of combating lurking feelings of depression or exhaustion. Sugary snacks are best avoided as they would raise your blood sugar levels too rapidly, with a bigger dip afterwards.

You could ask your partner – and perhaps friends and visitors – to make you some nutritious meals. Could he prepare some handy snacks first thing to help you eat enough through the day?

Healthy Eating in the Early Days

It's not always easy to eat well when you're struggling to get through a day spent learning how to care for your baby. Some nutritious snacks you could keep in the fridge or store cupboard are:

- Slices of cheese
- Bananas, avocados, apples, raw carrots, sticks of celery, dried fruit
- Rice cakes
- Low-fat yoghurt
- Popcorn – good for you but feels like a treat.

Aim for meals that can be prepared quickly. Here are some quick, nutritious ideas:

- Hot or cold pasta mixed with tinned tuna and fresh tomatoes
- Ham or cheese sandwiches on wholegrain bread
- Baked beans, scrambled eggs or sardines on toast
- A bowl of vegetable soup and a roll spread with butter
- Baked potato with cheese and pineapple or coleslaw.

If you're feeling a bit constipated after birth, you could try eating high-fibre cereals, prunes, figs and dried apricots. For flatulence or early day wind (common after a caesarean section), try peppermint tea or a drop of peppermint essence in some hot water. If you feel tired and irritable, and if you are getting mouth sores, you could boost your vitamin B levels with a Marmite sandwich on whole-grain bread, or a bowl of fortified breakfast cereal.

Foods to Avoid

There are no special foods or drinks for a breastfeeding mother. As for all busy mothers, a sensible diet is best. The Department of Health recommends that breastfeeding women in families with allergies should avoid peanuts, and it's also worth remembering that alcohol, caffeine and other drugs will pass into your breastmilk, so remember to tell your pharmacist and doctor that you're breastfeeding if you need any medication. You can now eat those foods you avoided in pregnancy, which could cause listeria or salmonella, such as soft cooked eggs, soft ripened cheeses and cook-chilled foods, as these bacteria cannot pass through breastmilk.

Please don't start to feel guilty if you also indulge in crisps or chocolates – you want to spend these early weeks enjoying your baby! However, if you can try to eat mostly healthy things it will help you feel more energetic and on top of things, and you are likely to return to your pre-pregnancy size sooner.

What about Toxins?

From time to time there are stories in the press about toxins in breast-milk, which come from exposure to pollution. In fact, all of us are exposed to these chemicals, including our babies in the womb, and it's just easier for scientists to measure them in breastmilk. Breastmilk is still better for your baby than formula milk, which will also contain toxins as cows are exposed to environmental pollution too. The best way to protect your baby is to ensure you have a nutritionally adequate diet, so that your own body will be more efficient at dealing with environmental toxins. If you smoke, have smoked recently or if you are exposed to cigarette smoke, then you may be deficient in vitamins B and C and possibly also in iron and zinc. Unrefined, wholemeal foods, vegetables and fruit will help to restore the balance.

Losing Weight

During pregnancy, you will have put on at least a stone in weight, perhaps two or even three. Obviously, some of your weight gain will be due to the baby, the placenta and the amniotic fluid, but the rest of the weight is stored as fat. Your body lays down these stores to make sure you have reserves to feed your baby. In the months after the birth, if you are breastfeeding and eating a sensible balanced diet when you are hungry, the fat will gradually break down and be used to nourish your baby. Crash dieting while you are breastfeeding is not sensible. Not only will you feel run down, but you may also release toxins stored in body fat into your bloodstream and therefore into your milk.

Some women swear they never lose weight while breastfeeding, but that it falls off as soon as they stop. Other women find they lose weight easily throughout the time they're breastfeeding. Many women will lose two to four pounds per month without even trying if they are breastfeeding exclusively. Because your body is burning up extra calories every day in the process of creating milk, you should lose weight if you continue to eat at your previous level. You may find you are ravenously hungry, or perhaps you find that your metabolism has slowed down and you won't lose weight until you have stopped. As long as you eat healthily when you are hungry, breastfeeding will help you burn off that fat, either now or in months to come.

If weight gain and your eating pattern has been a problem for you in the past, assume that they will continue to be so now. Be aware of what you eat, and stop eating when you feel full. You can maintain a sensible weight-reducing diet once breastfeeding is established, without affecting your milk supply. Talk to your health visitor or GP.

Now you are a mother, do you really want to look like a stick insect? Babies love to be cuddled, and a stick insect is not cuddly. Perhaps we shouldn't expect to be slender while nursing. Bumpy hips are useful to rest our babies on when we carry them. Even if you regain your pre-pregnancy weight, there is a good chance that your shape will have changed.

Your Questions Answered

Q Are there any foods that might upset my baby?

A People may tell you to avoid curries, garlic or onions, but if these really did give babies indigestion, babies fed on a Mediterranean or Indian diet would be crying continually. The truth is that some foods might upset some babies, so eat everything in moderation. If you suspect something has disagreed with your baby, then he is likely to suffer 12–24 hours later, with perhaps explosive, green nappies.

Q **Is it safe to exercise when you're breastfeeding?**

A Absolutely, but you don't need to rush off to the gym. Walking with a pushchair is great exercise. Find out about postnatal exercise classes in your area, through the NCT, YMCA or local leisure centre. As you will all be in the same boat, you won't need to splash out on expensive exercise clothes; probably everyone else will be in their maternity leggings. Do make sure, however, that you wear a good supportive bra to exercise in if you are breastfeeding.

> I do try and eat more healthily because of breastfeeding Soren – lots of veg and I take my vitamins but I have lots of treats too. I seem to be hungry all the time, and constantly having little snacks, but the weight doesn't go on.

Vic, mother to Esme (3 years) and Soren (3 months)

Myth or Fact?

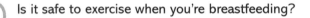

You need to Drink Milk to make Milk

Myth. After all, no other mammals need to drink milk to make milk! Adults in many other cultures never touch dairy products, yet their babies are breastfed.

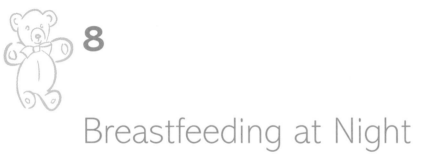

8

Breastfeeding at Night

Night feeds are probably one thing that all pregnant women and new mothers worry about, whether they intend to breastfeed or not.

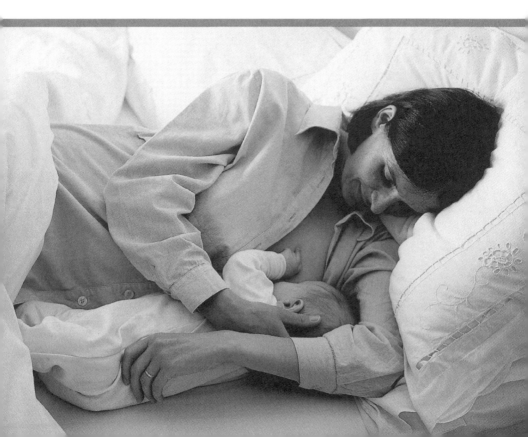

At first, neither you nor your baby will know what to expect, and the idea of having a routine or of getting a decent night's sleep might seem like an impossible dream. Don't worry – you will get there. In the meantime, try to enjoy these precious moments with your new baby rather than fretting about establishing a perfect schedule.

As you will have seen in Chapter 3, breastfeeding your baby whenever she seems hungry is important in those early weeks. She may well sleep between feeds; like you, she will be tired after the birth, so if you can nap at the same time you will start to regain your strength.

Why does your Baby need to Feed at Night?

Benefits for your Baby:

- Your baby needs milk at night because she simply can't store enough food during the day to keep her going.
- Breastfeeding at night is lovely and comforting, helping her get back to sleep.

Benefits for you:

- Breastfeeding at night in the early weeks helps your milk supply get established. The more you feed, the higher your prolactin levels, and therefore the more milk you will make.
- You may well find you wake frequently anyway to check your baby is OK. It's natural to worry about her when she is so little, and therefore breastfeeding gives you a cuddly time together.
- When you breastfeed at night, prolactin helps you get back to sleep: a big advantage over bottle-feeding. You probably found sleeping difficult in the weeks leading up to the birth. Maybe this was your body's way of preparing you for these disturbed nights! Now at least you have a great way of dozing off again.

Your baby is born not knowing the difference between day and night. Initially she drifts from deep sleep, through dozing to being wide awake, without understanding that we adults expect day and night to be different.

Although your baby has to feed during the night, you might also want her to learn to get back to sleep again quickly. It can help if you:

1 Avoid putting on a light. Use a night-light if you need to see what you are doing.
2 Try not to chat or interact with her if possible – low murmurs and gentle, soothing cuddles are best.
3 Don't change her nappy unless she is smelly, has a sore bottom, or has wet clothes.

How Feeding and Sleeping might Interact

All human beings rouse briefly several times during the night and mostly we go back to sleep without becoming aware of it. Once your baby is managing to go for a few hours between feeds, your rousing times might happen when she needs a feed. Many mothers find they 'tune into' their baby's sleep pattern. So even if you have to wake several times a night, it won't feel too bad if it coincides with your own sleep patterns. What mothers often find is that baby's waking is more of a problem when:

- her cycle disrupts yours
- she is difficult to settle
- her patterns change; perhaps she starts waking more frequently, or at different times. This is why it feels such a shock to be woken during the night after a couple of nights of sleeping through.

When your Baby might Sleep through the Night

Although babies do need to feed at night in the beginning, eventually night waking will become more about comfort and needing you to help her get back to sleep, than actually about hunger. Then she will be able to manage physically without so many night feeds, but it's not always easy to work out when this time arrives.

Rather than get hung up about what other people tell you 'ought' to happen, perhaps you could just think about what you and your family want. For instance, if you are finding night feeding OK, then you might be content to wait until she seems ready to sleep for longer. If, however, you feel like a zombie and that sleep deprivation is a form of torture, then it is time to cut down on night feeding!

Bearing in mind that your baby will wake every few hours anyway because all humans have cyclical sleep patterns, what you can do is help her get back to sleep at these points without feeding or waking you. If you always breastfeed her to sleep, then she may not be able to fall asleep without your breast. So the first step is to put her back in her cot after feeds, when she is warm and dozy but before she actually falls asleep.

Next you will want to cut down on the number of night feeds. It works best to drop one at a time. Initially you will need to help her get back to sleep without that feed. Try to become aware of when her cry means 'I am tired and want to sleep' or when it means something else, like 'I am hungry/cold/frightened' (*the next chapter looks at crying*). It is better if someone else can go and comfort her until she is used to doing without a breastfeed every time she wakes.

Where should your Baby Sleep?

The nearer your baby is to your bed, the easier and less disruptive it is to feed her in the early days. It's also safer for your baby to sleep in your room, as research shows there is an increased risk of cot death for babies who sleep in a separate room. Many parents start with their baby in a cot or Moses basket by the bed. While your baby's snuffling and snoring may disturb you, many mothers say they like being able to hear their baby breathe, and prefer to be woken by this than to lie awake worrying whether she is OK.

Breastfeeding at night can be easier if your baby is in bed with you. Once you both have the hang of feeding lying down (*see Chapter* 4) you will find that you barely wake up when she feeds, and that it's more restful than getting out of bed. In many cultures throughout the world and throughout history, babies have shared their parents' bed. In fact, we are in a minority expecting babies to sleep alone; many societies think our approach is barbaric.

Having said that, your baby is growing up into a culture where the norm, whether we like it or not, is to sleep alone. If you intend having another baby soon, it might feel like a double insult to your toddler to have her mummy cuddling a new baby *and* to have that baby take her place in bed.

You don't need to decide before your baby arrives whether to sleep with her or not. You might find it becomes obvious what's best once she's here. However, you and your partner need to talk about it, and it is important that you both feel happy about it. Although co-sleeping might not seem the norm, do be assured that far more people sleep with their babies, even in this country, than would otherwise appear.

Your Questions Answered

Q My baby seems to be waking more often now to feed; does this mean she needs solids?

A There are lots of reasons a baby might start waking more often in the night, but needing solids is rarely the answer – have a look ahead to Chapter 15 on introducing solids. Sometimes it is worth trying to breastfeed more during the day to make sure she is getting enough, but there may be other reasons why your baby isn't sleeping. It could be a change of some sort. An appetite or developmental spurt may make her restless and irritable. Some women find that after they return to work their baby feeds more often during the night. It is as if she's making up for your loss during the day, so you could view this as a positive step, if you can cope with the disturbed nights!

Q Is there any danger to my baby if she's in bed with us?

A It is recommended that you don't have the baby in your bed if you or your partner are under the influence of alcohol or drugs, or are extremely tired or if either of you smokes. You will also need to make sure that your baby is in no danger from overheating or suffocating under your pillow or quilt. There have been some cases of SIDS (Sudden Infant Death Syndrome, or cot death) where the parents were sleeping with their baby, but there are far more cases of cot death where the baby was in another room. In some cultures where nearly every baby shares their parents' bed, cot death is unknown. The thinking at the moment is that the baby is safer sleeping in a cot beside your bed in the same room for the first six months.

> Soren wakes up two or three times a night. He starts off in his little basket by the bed and I feed him around 10pm but when he wakes up again around 2am, I just bring him into bed with me, feed him and roll over. He stays there until morning. Miles, my partner, is on the sofa bed now because his snoring was keeping me awake! If Esme wakes up, she goes in with Miles – but mostly she sleeps through in her own bed.

Vic, mother of Soren (three months) and Esme (three years)

Myth or Fact?

All Babies should Sleep through the Night by Six Weeks

Myth. It takes many babies much longer than this to learn to maintain sleep for more than a few hours. If you are breastfeeding, however, your hormones will help you go straight off to sleep again. This is what makes the broken nights bearable. Sharing your bed or your bedroom with your baby will mean less disruption.

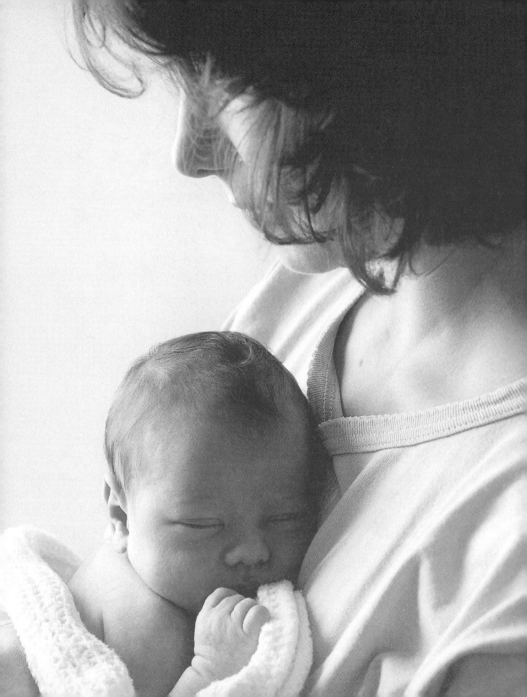

Part 4

Breastfeeding Problems

9

Crying, Colic and your Breastfeeding Baby

Every mother-to-be dreams of having a happy baby who rarely cries, but often the reality is different.

In the beginning, crying is the only means your baby has of letting you know something is wrong. Unfortunately, it is up to you to figure out precisely what. Although you may learn to identify your own baby's cry within a couple of days, it will take you much longer to recognize all the variations, and it's a challenge to learn what these different cries mean. A breastfeed will usually be the first thing to try, but there are other options too.

- Listen to your gut feeling – what do you think your baby needs?
- Most mothers try feeding first. Suckling is comforting, and you cannot overfeed a breastfed baby.
- Is he comfortable? Check his nappy, feel his abdomen to find whether he is too cold or hot.
- Is he in pain? This cry is quite distinctive – high-pitched, with breath holding in the middle, and will probably not stop even when you pick him up. If you are at all worried, ring your GP.
- If your baby is frightened or lonely, then he will be comforted when you pick him up. Cuddles and reassurance may be all he needs to settle, or you might carry him in a sling. Your baby loves to be rocked gently, as he was in your pelvis.
- A cry that means he feels tired, irritable or over-stimulated is hard to recognize, but it can be whiney or lower-pitched, with a rhythmic feel. Sometimes all the baby needs is to be given the chance to get himself to sleep, and unless the pattern of crying changes, it might be best to leave him, or perhaps give him a little stroke or other quiet, gentle reassurance.

Six-week Grizzle or 'Colic'

Everyone has heard of three-month colic, but no one really knows what it is. All we know is that 85 per cent of babies go through a grizzly stage, starting around three weeks of age, usually gone by twelve weeks, and with peak crying time at six weeks. With colic, crying is worst in the evenings when the baby draws his legs into his body as if he has cramp. Often he desperately wants to suck, but feeding doesn't seem to help, and crying can last two to three hours per day.

One theory says this six-week crying is 'jet lag'; your baby is reorganizing his internal workings to cope with a day/night cycle. Another theory claims the crying is caused by the way your baby's head was moulded during birth, or by a delayed shock from the delivery. Still others propose that your baby's fretfulness results from having too much information to process – this is why it occurs in the evening. Research suggests that this crying is a developmental stage, and nothing to do with parenting styles – so it's not your fault! Whatever the reason, it appears to be universal – babies from all cultures experience it, and it happens with first, second and later babies.

A baby that cannot be comforted is devastating. It is quite understandable that you will feel anxious and tense, but your baby will sense this, so try not to get drawn into his anxiety, but aim to handle him in a positive and confident way. Share the burden – make sure your family, friends and your partner take turns comforting him; he won't mind at this stage who's doing the cuddling. It can also be a great help to meet up with other new mums with colicky babies; ask your NCT branch or health visitor to put you in touch. If you feel you are losing your temper, then put your baby in his cot and walk away until you calm down, and ring someone like Serene (*see Appendix* 2) for help.

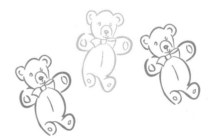

Is Feeding the Problem or the Solution?

Breast and bottle-fed babies suffer equally from colic, so switching feeding methods isn't the answer. Sucking is the most comforting thing your baby knows and it helps move gas along the intestine, so if he has a sore tummy your baby will want to feed even when he's not hungry.

It might be that your baby is getting mostly foremilk. If this is the case, he would be a bit gassy, often hungry, and he might have green, explosive nappies. To ensure that your baby is getting enough hind-milk, contact a breastfeeding counsellor who can check your baby's positioning. Some women who suspect that their colicky baby is getting too much foremilk find it helpful to allocate one breast for a certain time period, putting him back to the same breast every time he wants to feed. It is also generally good practice to let your baby decide when he has had enough rather than trying to limit his time at the breast.

Many mothers wonder if their baby is reacting to something in their breastmilk. This is a possibility, but hard to pinpoint as you need to exclude items from your diet for up to two weeks to see any difference, and then reintroduce them gradually as a 'trial'. Talk to a health professional, dietician or breastfeeding counsellor before going down this route. The commonest triggers are:

- Cow's milk proteins, especially if you or your partner have a family history of allergies. Excluding all dairy produce from your diet is difficult if you are used to it, and you need to make sure you have alternative sources of calcium.
- Caffeine, found in tea, coffee, cola and chocolate.

Bombarded Baby

If you think your baby is 'over-stimulated', then try creating a structured, early bedtime, perhaps with a soothing bath, a gentle cuddle and last feed *before* the miserable time starts. You could also cut down on stimulating events late afternoon.

Other Things to Try

There are lots of things you can try. It is best, however, to use only one strategy at a time, otherwise you won't know which is working:

- Babies under three months often like listening to 'white noise'. You can buy special 'womb noise' tapes, but the vacuum cleaner, washing machine or even un-tuned radio static can work just as well.
- Some babies like to be swaddled (see page 33), perhaps because it feels like the restricted space in the womb. Others like gentle singing or humming, especially with a head resting against his. You could also try lying down on your back in a darkened room with your baby lying on top of you. It's not safe to fall asleep on a sofa with your baby though.

Your Questions Answered

Q Are some babies just more demanding than others?

A Some babies are more 'high need' than others, and want to be held in close contact with their mums for seemingly hours on end. Denying a baby's need for contact won't make the need go away, but may create a frustrated baby. Babies have to learn that they're secure and loved, and a 'high need' baby may turn out to be more independent later once he knows he is loved.

Q Can alternative therapies help a crying baby?

A Alternative therapies don't always have research to back them up, but then there isn't a lot of research about colic anyway, and what exists is not definitive. Cranial osteopaths claim to have helped many babies with colic, particularly after an assisted birth with forceps or ventouse, which can give a baby a headache. They also claim to help babies born particularly quickly or by caesarean.

Q What about aromatherapy?

A Again, research evidence is not clear, and many essential oils are not suitable for babies. However, baby massage can soothe. Use only a simple vegetable oil such as olive or almond and slow stroking movements, keeping one hand in contact with his body at all times. Bathing your baby sometimes works, especially if you jump in too! Keep the bath temperature at body heat (not too hot), and make sure the bathroom is warm, with plenty of towels ready for you both to snuggle up in, as your baby will get chilled quickly.

Alasdair, our first baby, was breastfed and suffered from colic from two weeks until he was three months. He cried from around 6pm, carrying on some nights until 2 or 3am. It was devastating. I had this rosy picture of motherhood when I was pregnant, and reckoned my baby wouldn't cry. When he seemed so miserable and didn't care whether I was there or not, it was awful. I tried everything: cranial osteopathy, slings, constant feeding, drugs. My husband did his neck in carrying him over his shoulder for hours on end. Looking back, I think he was filling up on foremilk because I kept switching sides. We also weren't good at getting him to bed, and a consistent bedtime routine would have helped. We've done this with our other children, and they were fine, I am glad to say.

Caroline

Myth or Fact?

Picking your Baby up whenever He Cries will 'Spoil' Him

Myth. At this age your baby is incapable of manipulative behaviour; all he knows is that he has a need, and crying is his way of communicating that need to you.

10

Avoiding Problems

Breastfeeding is usually an enjoyable experience for both mother and baby, but it's disheartening if you encounter difficulties.

Many women who choose to breastfeed will get off to a good start and will enjoy it. For others, difficulties can make breastfeeding feel like a chore. As with any new undertaking, breastfeeding needs to be learnt, and everyone can make mistakes. Understanding what the common problems are and how to avoid them should help. Try not to ignore difficulties in the hope that they will go away, but tackle them as soon as they arise.

Sore Nipples

Many women have sensitive nipple skin for the first week after birth, and combined with the unfamiliar, strong sensation of your baby's feeding action, it can feel uncomfortable. As long as your nipples are not damaged or distorted in any way, it will quickly pass. When your baby latches on, wait for 30 seconds, and if you still feel uncomfortable, take your baby off your breast by inserting a clean finger into the corner of her mouth to break the suction, and try again. Practise relaxation at the beginning of the feed, and try to latch your baby on when she is just waking up, before she gets really hungry.

If your nipples become damaged, then feeding will be incredibly painful, although they will heal quickly. Now it is even more important to keep asking for help until you find someone who can show you a more comfortable position for holding the baby. Try to keep feeding your baby if you can, as you need to keep stimulating your nipples to maintain your supply. If the pain is worse on one side, it might help to start a feed off on the other side, and swap once your baby is feeding less hungrily. Alternatively, you could express milk to feed your baby as well as to keep your supply going.

It may be suggested that you use a nipple shield to prevent further damage and to protect your nipple, although suction through the nipple shield can open the cracks. If feeding does not feel possible without a shield, then this may be one option. The main problem, particularly with the 'Mexican Hat'-shaped nipple shields, is that using them may reduce your milk supply, and seems to alter your baby's sucking action. Many women find it hard to get rid of nipple shields afterwards – their babies seem to prefer the super-stimulation of this artificial nipple.

You might find it helps to use a pure, hypoallergenic lanolin ointment after every feed until your nipples heal. This ointment prevents scabs forming and keeps the nipple skin moist while it heals. Women also find it soothing. Pat your breasts dry before applying it. You don't need to remove it before the next feed. It's like putting lip salve on your lips if they were cracked.

It is miserable if you have sore nipples. Try to hang on to the fact that once you have tackled the cause of the problem, your nipples will get better very quickly. Most sore nipples are caused by problems with positioning and attachment, which is understandable; holding your baby the right way when you and she are all fingers and thumbs is hard. Have a look at Chapter 4, and get help from your midwife or breastfeeding counsellor. The NCT Breastfeeding Line 0870 444 8708 can also help.

Thrush

Another, less common cause of sore nipples is thrush (*Candida albicans*), a fungal infection. Consider this if you have had thrush during pregnancy, are prone to thrush or if you or your baby have recently taken antibiotics. Thrush causes nipple pain, and sometimes deep breast pain; your nipple skin may look pinker than usual and shiny, and your baby may have white patches on her tongue or in her mouth. Women describe the pain as sharp and stabbing, like needles, and it often continues between feeds. Nipples can be sensitive to cold, and water on the skin is unbearable. It is important that both you *and your baby* are treated by your GP or pharmacist with anti-fungal medication, even if only one of you has symptoms, otherwise you can re-infect each other. Talk to a breastfeeding counsellor about the current, recommended treatments.

Sore Breasts

When your baby is feeding, your breasts 'let down' milk; hormones cause little muscles high up in your breasts to contract, squeezing milk down towards your nipples where the baby can get it. Some women are unaware of this; others find it a strange, almost tickly feeling, but a few will find it painful. It should quickly pass; try to relax through it.

Two to five days after the birth, your milk 'comes in', which happens whether you are breastfeeding or not. Your breasts become hot, swollen and uncomfortable, and it can be hard for your baby to latch on. We call this 'engorgement' but your breasts are not full of milk; they are swollen with excess fluid due to an increased blood supply. This usually passes within 24 hours; in the meantime, feeding your baby frequently will help. Many women find that applying warm water to the breasts before a feed, or ice cold flannels afterwards, brings relief.

If your breasts become engorged when your baby is older, perhaps because she's missed a feed, you can express some milk to relieve the discomfort, otherwise you could develop a blocked duct, or even mastitis. As your ducts are always filling up with milk, your breasts will vary in size and shape all the time, and lumps will appear occasionally. These should never last long because whenever your baby feeds, she normally drains them. If you have a lump that seems persistent, it may be the beginning of a blocked duct, especially if it feels tender. Feed your baby with her lower jaw as near to the lump as possible; if it occurs on the outer side of your breast, for instance, try feeding underarm on that side. You might also find it helpful to massage the lump gently towards your nipple while your baby is feeding.

If you are getting recurring blocked ducts, think about where on your breasts they happen, and what therefore might be restricting the flow of milk:

- Does your bra fit well?
- Is something restricting your milk flow during a feed, such as your hand or your baby's hand?

Mastitis

Most women have heard of mastitis, but don't worry – not many end up getting it. If you are unlucky enough to develop mastitis, you will feel fluey, may have a temperature, and your breasts will be sore. Try to rest and drink plenty of fluids. It is important to keep feeding your baby, as stopping breastfeeding will make the problem worse. Usually mastitis results from insufficient drainage of the breast – from delayed feeds, attachment which is not quite right, blocked ducts or untreated engorgement. If you can correct the problem, the mastitis will ease, and will not require medication.

Your GP may prescribe antibiotics but most cases of mastitis are not caused by infection, so antibiotics here are preventative. However, in a few rare cases, mastitis does result from an infection which can lead to an abscess and will require antibiotics. Alternatively, your GP may prefer to prescribe an anti-inflammatory drug to reduce the inflammation. Neither of these will harm your baby, though antibiotics may upset her tummy, and you will then need to watch out for thrush.

If you can identify why you got mastitis, you can probably prevent it happening in the future, so talk it through with a breastfeeding counsellor.

It may sound as though breastfeeding is all problems, problems. Do remember that most women encounter few, if any, difficulties, and no one experiences all of them!

While you are breastfeeding it will be impossible for you to examine your breasts for lumps, as these will come and go all the time. When you stop breastfeeding, however, you should start to do regular breast examinations, especially if you have never done so before. Ask your GP or practice nurse for help if you don't know what to do, but remember that nine out of ten breast lumps are not cancer, and that breastfeeding will help to protect you against this disease.

Your Questions Answered

 I have sore nipples, and after feeding they are chafed.

 Your nipple is probably rubbing against your baby's hard palate. Your baby needs to open her mouth really wide, and you should hold her so that your nipple is aiming at the roof of her mouth.

Q **My baby seems to find feeding almost painful, and pulls away and cries. As my nipples are also sore, this feels excruciating.**

A It sounds as if you could both have thrush – this would make feeding painful for your baby as her mouth will be sore. You should seek appropriate treatment from your GP.

> I felt sore at the beginning with both of them. This pain lasted just over a week, but once it settled down it was fine. I really enjoyed feeding them. However, I got mastitis when Victoria was three months old. I felt awful, and was convinced I was going to have to give up. My GP was really helpful. She came to visit me at home and reassured me that I didn't need to stop. I carried on and it didn't happen again.

Maggie, mother of Victoria and David

Myth or Fact?

Women with Fair Skin are more likely to get Sore Nipples

No, it's definitely a **myth** that fair-skinned women are more likely to get sore nipples. Just like all women, they may feel uncomfortable for the first week, while they get used to breastfeeding. If the baby is positioned correctly, she can feed for as long as both mother and baby want.

11
Breastfeeding Premature Babies and Twins

Sometimes special circumstances make breastfeeding harder. These include multiple birth, an illness or disability, or being born prematurely.

Premature Babies

To give birth to a baby prematurely is always a shock and looking after your baby in a special care baby unit (sometimes called a neonatal unit or SCBU for short) can be distressing. Instead of lying in your arms where he should be, your baby will need to spend time in an incubator surrounded by machinery.

If your baby is very small or unwell, he won't have strong sucking or swallowing reflexes yet, so to give the benefits of breastmilk, you'll need to express your milk by hand or with a pump. At first, your baby may need to be fed using a naso-gastric tube. This is a tube that goes through the baby's nose and into his stomach and is left in place, with sticking plaster over his nose, between feeds. Sometimes the milk is given as a continuous feed with the help of a small electric pump, which makes it possible for your baby to get his food without expending energy.

When he is ready, he can progress to feeding from a cup or bottle, but even while he is still at the tube-feeding stage you can cuddle him close so that he can lick or nuzzle your breast in a breastfeeding position.

And when your baby is ready to try breastfeeding properly, you can put him to your breast with the tube in place. If your baby is not strong enough to get all his nutritional requirements at the breast, he can be supplemented later, or at the same time, through the tube.

Expressing your milk is not a lot of fun; it's hard work and you'll need all the support and encouragement you can get – but it's worth it. Many mothers find it really comforting to provide breastmilk for their pre-term baby because it's the one thing they alone can do.

Breastmilk is especially suited to pre-term babies because of their immature digestive systems. It contains factors that protect them from infection and allergy, and research has even shown that the milk from mothers of premature babies is higher in protein than the breastmilk of mothers of full-term babies. Breastmilk also protects babies from the very dangerous necrotising enterocolitis.

Expressing Breastmilk

The most common method of expressing milk for a pre-term baby is with an electric breast pump. If you can start pumping as soon as possible after the birth, you will be able to give your baby more of your valuable colostrum, although you may not be in a fit state to even think about it.

You may, in fact, find hand-expressing easier than pumping, so ask a midwife or breastfeeding counsellor to show you how. Gently massaging your breasts before you start and rinsing out a flannel in warm water and placing it against your breasts can help the milk to flow. It can often help to look at your baby, or a photo of your baby, while expressing.

It's best to express your milk frequently and regularly – little and often is best, say every three hours for 10 minutes, or more frequently. You could aim for six to eight times over 24 hours, including at least one session at night.

If you find that expressing is slow, most electric breast pumps allow dual pumping. Expressing from both breasts at the same time is more efficient and gives your breasts maximum stimulation. Remember that every drop of milk your baby receives is a bonus, so try not to worry if the volume seems small.

It helps to get into the routine of using the pump as soon as possible in the hospital. When you go home, you can hire a breast pump through the National Childbirth Trust, from your local breastfeeding counsellor or via the NCT Breastfeeding Line (0870 444 8708). The NCT will also be able to give you more support and information if your baby is in special care.

There's more information on expressing breastmilk in Chapter 13, and organizations you can contact for help are listed in Appendix 2.

Cup Feeding

Babies born as early as 32 weeks can be fed from a cup (a small plastic medicine cup, in fact). Premature babies tend to 'lap' the milk in this way. This method can also help with feeding a baby with a cleft palate.

Babies who have difficulty breastfeeding, for any reason, are often fed breastmilk via a bottle, and then later have to get used to the different sucking style of breastfeeding. Many find it hard, and so their mothers sometimes resort to bottle-feeding formula. The advantage of a cup over a bottle is that your baby won't have to make the difficult switch from bottle to breast, and babies usually enjoy it.

How to Cup Feed

- Hold the baby upright and preferably swaddled to prevent his hands knocking the cup and spilling the precious colostrum or breastmilk.
- Have the cup as full as possible but don't worry if there is only a small quantity.
- Tip the cup so that the rim is directed towards the baby's upper gum and the level of milk is touching the baby's lips.
- Wait for the baby to take the milk. Do not pour milk into the baby's mouth. The action varies between lapping and sucking.
- Keep the cup and the level of milk in place between feeding bursts. (This is nothing like teaching a toddler to drink from a cup when a mouthful is given at a time, the cup removed and the dribbles scooped up.)
- The baby will pace the feed and will not carry on once he has had enough.

Kangaroo Care

Parents may have difficulty coming to terms with a baby who looks nothing like the full-term infant they imagined. Some may feel safer cutting off their emotions rather than risking bonding with a sick new-born, but this can lead to feelings of guilt.

'Kangaroo care' is the name of a very effective method of keeping premature babies warm outside an incubator. It has been shown to make bonding and breastfeeding easier. Your baby is simply placed in a nappy against your bare chest, between your breasts, and both of you are then covered up. This gives your baby skin-to-skin contact and easy access to your breasts. A study at Hammersmith Hospital in London showed that babies who had even small amounts of kangaroo care put on weight more rapidly and were allowed home more quickly than those being looked after in standard intensive care – so do mention kangaroo care to the SCBU nurses caring for you and your baby.

Breastfeeding Twins

With one baby, it may take time to become confident at breastfeeding because you're both learning, but when you have twins it can be even more daunting. One brilliant thing to hang on to is that your body is capable of producing enough milk to feed twins, or even triplets, as long as you don't try to limit the amount they feed in the early days. Twins especially benefit from breastmilk's protective properties, as they might be pre-term or have had a difficult entry into the world.

The First Few Weeks with Breastfed Twins

- Twins are usually smaller than singletons, and thus getting positioning right can be harder. They will also tire more easily and may feed little and often. Make sure someone is there to help you latch the babies on until you feel totally confident.
- If your babies are born prematurely, they will probably need tube feeding at first. Any breastmilk you express for them will be valuable.
- Babies who are born around 37 weeks, as many twins are, don't usually have a mature suckling reflex. They may latch on but then won't milk the breast. This will pass, and in the meantime, cup feeding your babies (see page 78) will ensure they quickly adapt to the breast when they're ready.
- You might have had a caesarean, which makes holding two babies difficult. The underarm hold is useful, or you can feed one baby at a time lying down.
- Remember that breastfeeding will save you time in the long run.

Some mothers who are breastfeeding twins feel permanently hungry. The problem can be finding time to eat enough to satisfy your appetite when you have two tiny babies to care for. Perhaps your family can provide plenty of nutritious snacks and meals. If you find you aren't able to sit down for a full meal, you could eat a healthy snack or have a drink every hour or so. You may well feel hungry in the night too, so have some sandwiches ready.

Feeding Twins Together or Separately – which way Works Best?

Although it's possible to feed twins simultaneously, it takes practice. In the early days, therefore, you may prefer feeding one at a time, though it may feel as if you never do anything but breastfeed!

The advantage of feeding separately is that you have time with each baby individually. However, the second one may be crying with hunger while you feed the first. Perhaps someone else could comfort him, and when he's a bit older he could sit in a cradle chair and you could chat to him while you finish feeding the first baby.

If you would like to feed both babies simultaneously, you will eventually get adept at scooping up one baby with each hand. It's important that each baby latches correctly as you will have no spare hand to readjust things. Different-sized babies often have different appetites, so one may finish first. You could pat him across your knee while you finish feeding the other.

Options for feeding together:

- babies' heads together on a pillow on your lap, with their feet on more pillows sticking out to your side – alternatively you could use one V-shaped pillow
- one baby in traditional position, the other underarm
- both in traditional position, one immediately behind the other.

Your Questions Answered

Q Is it better to assign one breast to each twin?

A Twins often do have a preferred breast, and if you give each baby its own side, each breast will produce the amount that baby needs. However, if your babies are different weights, or if one is not well, it's worth swapping sides to get the bigger baby to stimulate the other breast.

Q I want the babies to get into a routine, but I've heard you should let the babies feed whenever they ask. What should I do?

A You have three options. Firstly, you could feed the babies whenever they want – demand feeding. It's only for a short time in the babies' lives, and if you have people to help you in other ways, it's the best way of regulating your milk supply. Secondly, you could try modified baby-led feeding. Let one baby wake spontaneously and feed, but then deliberately wake the second to feed. This will work if the babies don't have wildly different appetites. Thirdly, you can impose a feeding schedule on them but it is better to wait until they are a few weeks old and established breastfeeders.

Phil and I were completely thrown by Thomas and James's arrival. We had twins in the family, but a long way back, so it was a complete surprise. Luckily my mum lives close by and was happy to help. That first year, leaving the house was a big challenge; it would be nearly lunchtime before I had finished feeding and changing them. Bathtimes were a nightmare until they could both sit up. Breastfeeding was enjoyable though; I used to feed them together with one under each arm, and I carried on for eight months.

Kate

Myth or Fact?

You must Eat and Drink lots of Special Food to make enough Milk for Twins

Myth. Your body can make breastmilk from whatever you eat. It is best to eat to appetite and drink to thirst. You don't need to eat more than you feel like. However, it is important that you don't skip meals, and try to eat snacks which are nutritious – have a banana or a sandwich rather than a chocolate biscuit!

12

Babies who Bite

Clamping your jaw shut is a common human reaction to pain. Therefore, if your baby bites, she doesn't mean to hurt you, but might herself be reacting instinctively to pain.

There are many reasons why a breastfeeding baby might bite. If she has a sore mouth, for instance, through teething, thrush or mouth ulcers, breastfeeding can remind her or even make it feel worse. Occasionally, a baby might bite because of sudden pain elsewhere in her body.

Some mothers wean their babies when they think they're about to produce teeth, but breastfeeding with teeth is normal and natural. Your baby's teeth may appear at any age – on average the first breaks through at around six months – but many babies remain toothless for much longer and a few babies are even born with teeth.

It's impossible, in fact, for a baby to bite with her first teeth when she's actually breastfeeding as her tongue covers her lower gum ridge – where the first teeth break through. In order to bite, she would need to pull her tongue back to expose her teeth – which she can't do while latched on. However, teething is one cause of mouth pain, and therefore your baby might do some teething-related biting as her first tooth erupts.

The First Time She Bites

Newly emerged teeth are sharp, and if these graze or even fasten onto your breast, the chances are you will scream or shout! Your strong reaction might shock your baby so much that she won't do it again. Some particularly sensitive babies can be startled or even frightened by a strong reaction and then refuse the breast. The more usual reaction to your scream, however, is that your baby feels curious, and repeats the bite to see if it works again – a bit like experimenting with a push button toy or rattle. If this happens, try to stay calm and quiet, but stop feeding her, make eye contact, and give her a firm 'no'.

If Biting Continues

There is still no need to wean unless you want to; being aware of the cause of biting in your own case, and satisfying your baby's need to bite in other ways, is likely to resolve the problem quickly. Most mothers find that breastfeeding continues to be a positive experience once the biting episodes stop.

If your baby has sore gums, she may want to bite down to relieve the soreness. You could try giving her a cold teething ring to chew on before you feed her. While over-the-counter teething gels can soothe your baby, don't use them before you feed as they can numb the baby's tongue and might also numb your areola, making feeding difficult for both of you. Some teething gels can irritate sensitive nipple skin too. If you want to use one of these preparations, it would be better to apply it after a feed.

A Number of other Reasons why your Baby might Bite:

- Frustration. Perhaps your let-down reflex is not happening quickly enough; it can be slow to start if you are upset or distracted. Perhaps your supply has decreased, especially if your baby is on solids and feeding less often. If you think this might be the reason for biting, see if you can get your milk flowing before she starts to feed.
- Play bites. Sometimes older babies bite because they're not really interested in feeding at that moment. If your baby is biting after playing around, it might be better to cut out comfort feeds until the biting episodes have stopped.
- The flavour of your milk has changed. Your changing hormones can affect the taste of your milk – after ovulation, during a period or during pregnancy. Less commonly, flavour changes after exercise, if you have an infection, or perhaps simply because you have eaten something different.
- Some babies bite at the end of a feed when they fall asleep. Watch for the slowing down and weakening of her jaw movements, and remove her before she dozes off.
- Some babies like to take the nipple with them when they are distracted and turn their heads! Keep your finger ready to break suction quickly in case she turns her head.
- Biting could be about trying to get your attention. It might be that for a while you will need to make an effort to keep focused on your baby during feeds – maintain eye contact, touch and talk to her. You will then be able to spot when she is about to bite you.

If your baby looks as though she is about to bite, put your little finger into the corner of her mouth, to come between her gums. She may then bite your finger rather than breast. If you try to pull her off while she's biting, you will only damage yourself. Watch for the tightening of her jaw before she bites down, and quickly take her off. You might need to give shorter feeds in general until this phase has passed.

Strategies to stop your baby biting:

- Say 'no' firmly and look her in the eye with displeasure. Stop the feed. She needs to associate biting with losing the breast.
- If she persists, put her on the floor for a short time immediately after she bites. Most babies will dislike this separation and hopefully will come to associate it with biting.
- For a persistent biter, be positive when she doesn't bite. Give her lots of hugs, kisses and praise.
- Give her your complete attention while feeding.
- Learn to recognize when she is finishing.
- Don't feed her unless she is really hungry.
- Take her off if she is falling asleep.
- Give her an acceptable teething object.

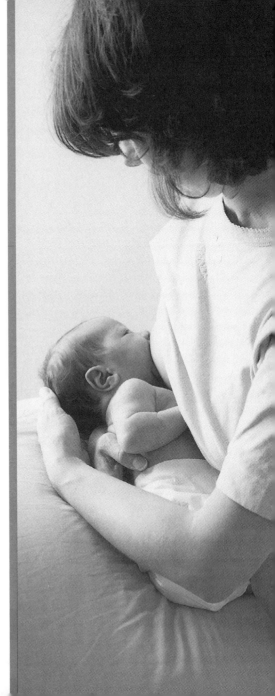

Your Questions Answered

 My baby is rejecting the breast, but I don't think she is really ready to wean. What can I do?

A If you have been breastfeeding successfully for a few months, and your baby suddenly rejects you, don't feel you have to give up. It could be a temporary set-back, with several possible reasons:

1 Your baby might be under the weather – an ear infection, or teeth coming through would make breastfeeding painful for her. Try expressing and feeding her your milk in a cup until she feels better.
2 The taste of your breastmilk might have changed. When you first ovulate, or if you have taken up exercise again, your milk can taste different.
3 Babies are very sensitive to smell, so think about whether you have changed your washing powder, deodorant, or have a new perfume – this could put her off.
4 When babies reach about four to six months of age, they love to look around and can easily be distracted by activities or noise. You may have to retire to a quiet, darkened room. Remember, though, feeds will naturally get shorter at this time as your baby is a very efficient feeder, and five minutes may be all she needs to fill up.

Things that may Help:

- Keep calm – remember, your baby is not rejecting *you*.
- Talk to your baby – reassure her that you are still there for her.
- Try skin-to-skin contact, which can be comforting even without breastfeeding.

- Offer her a feed when she is sleepy or even asleep.
- Change the way you hold your baby – if she has ear- or toothache this may help.

Greg started biting the nipple when he was about eight months old and his first two teeth were coming through. If I screamed and yanked him off, he would laugh. This was a great game! I found the only way to deal with him was to take him off, say 'no' very firmly, and sit him on the floor for a few minutes. Is it a coincidence that his biting tailed off when his four front teeth were through?

Fiona

Myth or Fact?

You need to Prepare your Nipples for Breastfeeding before your Baby is Born

Myth. It makes no difference to the experience of breastfeeding.

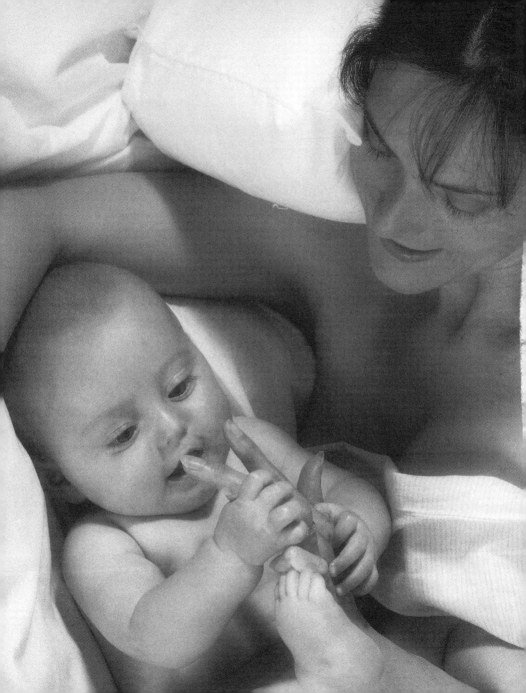

Part 5

Moving On

13

Combined Feeding

You will almost certainly need to introduce bottles if you are returning to work early, but in any case you may want to know that someone else can always feed your baby.

Your baby does not have to 'learn' to bottle-feed. Many babies pass happily from breastfeeding to using a cup as part of the family meal, without ever going through a stage of taking a bottle. Even if you are intending to return to work, your baby can by-pass having a bottle. At six months, babies can usually drink from a beaker.

Don't let anyone pressurize you to introduce bottles if you don't want to – such as a granny who wants to 'have a go' at feeding your baby, or a friend who wants you to 'get back to normal'. Within a short time it will get easier to leave your baby, and you might prefer to wait until then, rather than having to complicate your life with bottles at this stage. If you are worried about breastfeeding when you are out and about, talk to other mothers who have done it. More and more places welcome breastfeeding mothers, from supermarkets to libraries, as well as shops and cafés. Practise at home, so that you can breastfeed discreetly, without anything showing.

If, however, you do need to leave your baby with other people from an early age for whatever reason, you will also be faced with the decision of what to feed him – expressed breastmilk (EBM) or formula. You may prefer to give him EBM, especially if your family has a history of allergies, such as eczema, asthma or peanut allergy, and you want to avoid giving formula (*see Chapter* 1). You can also combine breastfeeding and formula if you find it difficult to express.

In Chapter 3, you saw that your milk supply operates on the principle of supply and demand. This means that if your baby has a bottle, he'll take less of your milk and so your supply will decrease. Once breastfeeding is well established, your supply will be harder to disrupt, but you will still not be able to miss feeds without discomfort. Expressing your milk at times when you would normally be giving a feed, but are temporarily away from your baby, is a good idea.

Rejecting the Breast

Some babies reject the breast if introduced to bottle teats before breastfeeding is happily established. This might happen because the large teat is a bigger stimulus for the baby. It can be hard work to coax the baby back to breastfeeding. Although there is not good research evidence on this, 'nipple confusion' seems less likely to occur once breastfeeding is established, so if your baby has to be fed artificially before then, it's probably better if he can be fed by cup, spoon or syringe. Ask your midwife, breastfeeding counsellor or health visitor about special baby cups, and how to use them, and look back at the section on cup feeding pre-term babies in Chapter 11.

Rejecting the Bottle

Sometimes babies will also refuse bottles. Some things to try:

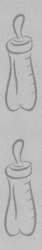

- Ask someone else – such as your partner, or your childminder if you are returning to work – to give the bottle. Your baby will not expect a breastfeed, and may be more willing to accept a bottle from them. It can help for you to leave the room completely.
- Try a different temperature – some babies will only accept milk at the same temperature as breastmilk, while others will take a bottle of cool milk.
- Experiment with different teats, and try warming them with hot water first.
- You may feel less pressured if you introduce the bottle about two weeks before you actually have to leave your baby. This will also give you time to experiment with different teats.

Expressing Breastmilk

If your baby only feeds from one breast at each feeding, you can express from the other breast, either by hand or using a breast pump you can operate with one hand. If he has long gaps between feeds (three hours or more) you can try expressing by hand or with a pump, in between feeds. Alternatively, you can express what is left after your baby has finished a feed. You'll need to experiment to find the best time and the best method for you. You'll find expressing gets easier with practice.

Getting Ready

Before you start, there are several things you can do to help your milk flow:

- Try to be as comfortable and relaxed as possible.
- Have your baby, or a photograph of your baby, close by.
- Have a warm bath or shower, or lay warm flannels on your breast.
- Gently stroke your breast towards the nipple.

Hand Expressing

- Hold your breast, with your thumb on top and your fingers underneath, so that your little finger is against your ribcage, and your first finger and thumb are opposite each other, making a big 'C' shape round your breast.
- Your milk comes from deep within your breast, so your finger and thumb need to be well away from your nipple, back behind your areola.
- Squeeze your thumb and first finger gently together, hold and release, and keep doing this without changing the position of your fingers, until you see some drops of milk appearing. This may take a few minutes.
- Some women find this more effective if they gently push their whole hand back, towards the ribcage, before they squeeze.
- If the flow of milk slows, you can move your hand round, keeping that 'C', so that you are 'milking' a different section of your breast.
- You can swap from side to side to increase the amount of milk expressed.

Using a Breast Pump

All pumps work by drawing the milk through your nipple into a steril-ized container. There are hand pumps and electric (battery and/or mains) pumps. You are really only likely to need a pump if you are returning to work early, if you are likely to be going out a lot, or if you or your baby are ill, otherwise hand expressing is just as efficient and is cost-free.

Storing Expressed Breastmilk (EBM)

EBM keeps well if refrigerated or frozen. It will last for at least 24 hours stored in the coldest part of the fridge (at 4 °C, 39 °F – usually the back or the bottom, NOT the door). Freezing only causes minor changes to the nutrients and anti-infective properties. Frozen EBM stored in a sep-arate freezer is best used within three months, but place it in the back, not the bottom.

You will need to freeze EBM in sterile containers. You may prefer to buy special EBM polybags as they have no harmful chemicals. Label and date the bag, and then pour the milk straight into it from the pump container. You can pop the bag straight into baby's bottle when you need to use it.

Chilled expressed milk can be added to milk which is already frozen, as long as you don't add more than half as much again. As milk will expand on freezing, don't fill containers to the top.

When feeding EBM to your baby, use fresh first and the oldest batch of frozen next. The fat in EBM often separates – simply give it a good shake. Milk defrosted in the fridge will keep for 24 hours. However, you can thaw milk quickly by standing the container in hot water, but you must use immediately. You can heat EBM in a bowl of hot water – don't heat it directly in a pan or microwave it, as this will destroy some nutritional benefits. Microwaves heat unevenly and hot spots could scald a baby. Milk does not have to be at body heat – babies don't mind it cool or at room temperature.

You can either use chemicals or heat to sterilize equipment. You need to wash and rinse bottles and teats immediately after use so that the film of milk doesn't harden. Then you can boil them, in which case they must be completely submerged and kept boiling for at least 10 minutes. The same principle of heating to destroy germs works in the microwave or baby steamer, and will take less time. Chemical sterilizers come with instructions about how long to submerge the bottles and teats, and it is recommended that the sterilizing fluid is changed at least every 24 hours.

Your Questions Answered

Q Should I give my baby a bottle of formula last thing at night to help him sleep?

A It might work, it might not. Bottle-fed babies do sometimes go longer at night between feeds, probably because formula milk is less digestible so it sits in the baby's tummy for longer. Once you substitute a bottle-feed for a breastfeed, the milk you have available at this time will go down. Introducing a bottle before your baby is really well established at the breast and you both feel breastfeeding is a doddle, may cause difficulty.

Q Which kind of breast pump do you recommend?

A It depends on how often you need to express. Hand pumps are cheap, portable and quiet. Avoid 'breast relievers' (with a rubber bulb), as these cannot be properly sterilized. Cylinder or lever mechanisms work well, but any pump requiring you to squeeze something will be very tiring. Battery or electric pumps are quick and effective, but make a noise and are more expensive. Try hiring one to begin with and shop around.

When I went back to work, I was happy with my hand pump. I used it at work twice a day for about 15 to 20 minutes at a time. I was lucky because I was working in a hospital and I could find places to slip into where I could express in peace. I used two sterilized bottles which I put in the fridge, and the milk was still cold when I got home.

Sarah

Myth or Fact?

Breastfeeding and Bottle-feeding cannot be mixed

Myth. You can mix breast and bottle, although it's best to wait until your baby is several weeks old before introducing bottles, as before this time it can affect your milk supply and confuse your baby.

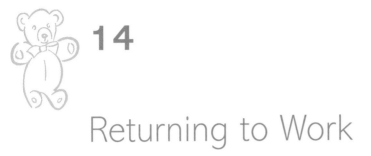

14

Returning to Work

Women have always worked and breastfed. Now that we travel further to workplaces where babies are not welcome, it has become more difficult. Yet with careful planning, breastfeeding is still possible, even if you will be apart from your baby most of the day.

Returning to work can be a terrible wrench. Continuing to breastfeed may feel really important: a way of nurturing your baby even when you are not there. Of course, your breastmilk will be protecting her in a very real way when you are apart, as the antibodies will help to defend her against other people's germs.

Even if you find you can't continue to feed when you are back at work, remember that breastfeeding even for a short time is better for both of you than not breastfeeding at all.

How much Milk will my Baby Need?

How much breastmilk your baby needs when you return to work will depend on her age. Breastmilk is all the food your baby needs for the first six months. If your baby is younger, she will be entirely dependent on milk, while an older baby will also need some milk feeds during a full working day. Your options are therefore:

- leaving expressed breastmilk (EBM) for your baby when you are not there
- combining breastmilk and formula milk.

Once your baby is over six months, she will be having some solids and will be able to manage longer without breastfeeds. If you are working short hours, you could feed her when you drop her off and as soon as you return. If you have a childminder, perhaps she could encourage your baby to have a late afternoon nap, waking to find you there, ready to feed her. However, you could also leave some frozen EBM for emergencies.

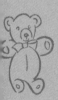

Some mothers arrange childcare near their workplace, so they can pop out during the day to breastfeed. While this may work for you, remember that your baby will only need breastfeeding during working hours for a relatively short time, and it might not be worth gearing childcare around this. Consider what the travelling would be like with a toddler before you make any decision.

Combining Breastfeeding with Formula Feeding

It is perfectly possible to breastfeed your baby only while you are with her and let a childminder or carer give her formula while you are at work. It may be that expressing milk at work would be difficult, or your job is long and stressful, and you don't feel able to provide fully for your baby's milk needs. Combined feeding – mixing breastmilk and formula milk – is still much better for your baby than stopping breastfeeding altogether (*see Chapter* 13).

You will need to cut out breastfeeds gradually, some time before returning. If you wean too quickly, you may get mastitis. It takes about three to seven days for your breasts to adjust to missing one feed. Ideally, you can drop one feed a week. Each time you miss a feed, your breasts will fill, and you should express off just enough milk to feel comfortable, without 'emptying' your breast. Once your breast no longer fills, you can move on to dropping the next feed.

Leaving Expressed Breastmilk for your Baby

You may want your baby to drink only your breastmilk, especially if you have a family history of allergies, eczema and asthma. You will need to talk it through beforehand with your childminder, nanny or nursery. They will need to feel confident about storing and handling EBM. Your employer or personnel department will also need to be aware of your arrangements, so that facilities for expressing at work can be provided, if they do not exist already.

It may be useful to talk through your options with a breastfeeding counsellor or other working mothers who have breastfed, to help choose the best method for you.

Before you return, discuss with your employer how expressing breast-milk could fit in to your working day. Find out how other women at your workplace managed, or talk to one of the organizations listed in Appendix 2 about how to approach your employer.

What is unlikely to work is trying to express secretly! You have a right to facilities for expressing and you will need somewhere clean and private (NOT the toilet) to express. Electric and battery pumps make some noise, and you need to be relaxed for the pump to work anyway, so it is likely to be essential that you have some guaranteed privacy.

You will also need to be able to store EBM safely until you can transfer it to your fridge or freezer or your childminder's. A fridge at work is ideal. Make sure the EBM is clearly labelled, as you don't want it to end up in your colleagues' tea! If a safe fridge is not available, you can keep EBM in a well-insulated cool box with ice packs for a few hours, except in very hot weather. You will need a cool box to transport EBM home from work at the end of the day.

Even with the most understanding of employers, you will probably feel some pressure to express quickly. A photo of your baby or a piece of clothing which smells of her can help get your milk flowing more quickly. 'Think milk' – imagine the milk flowing and it usually will.

Your working lifestyle will probably have to change from what it was 'pre-baby'. You will feel better if you eat well at work, even if you previously skipped meals. Don't miss your lunch to express! You need to look after yourself to look after your baby.

1　Decide whether you prefer to breastfeed fully, or combine formula and breast. Talk it over with a breastfeeding counsellor, your child-carer and your employer.

2　A few weeks before returning to work, you can start building up a store of expressed breastmilk (EBM). It is difficult to know how much she will need, so overestimate if you can. A rough guide is 2.5 oz of milk for each pound of baby's weight in 24 hours (or 125ml per kg). So, for example, a 10 lb baby might take 25 oz milk in 24 hours. Aim to have a few days' supply in hand when you start back at work and you can top up supplies thereafter with milk you express at work.

3　Three weeks to go – if you are opting for combined feeding, you will need to start dropping breastfeeds and replacing them with formula. Remember to drop only one feed at a time.

4　Two weeks to go – now is the time to stop expressing extra milk. Expressing builds up your supply, and you will need to tail this off so you are not producing masses at work. You need to introduce your baby to a bottle now if you have not done so already.

5　One week to go – a trial run is a good idea. Leave your baby for a couple of hours with your childminder so you can iron out difficulties beforehand.

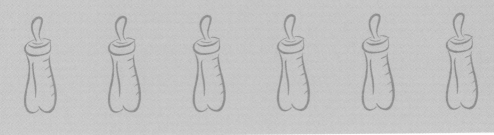

Your First Week at Work

Dark, patterned clothes are a good idea to start with to hide any signs of leaking. Choose tops that lift up or clothes that open at the front for expressing and for feeding your baby when you meet up at the end of the day.

If you have problems with leaking, press your elbows firmly against the outer margins of your breast. This will slow down the flow. It is worth taking a spare top for emergencies. Even if your baby is having formula while you are at work, you may still need to express off small amounts until your supply settles down.

Your Questions Answered

Q **I am returning to work early; is it worth starting breastfeeding at all?**

A Some mothers have to return to work before the statutory time, and wonder whether breastfeeding is worth doing at all. However long or short a time you feed your baby yourself, you will be giving her an invaluable start – have another look at Chapter 1. In fact, when you return to work, you could express milk for your baby to drink while you are away, or you could do combined feeding – your baby breastfeeds at nights and weekends, and has formula while you work. This is still a healthier option than no breastmilk at all. It's also a great way to relax and reconnect with your baby at the end of your working day.

Q How soon before I go back should I introduce a bottle?

A If you know you need to get your baby used to a bottle, it's generally better to wait until breastfeeding is established, but not leave it so long that your baby is unwilling to try anything new. Somewhere between three and six weeks after the birth often works well. Many women who intend to return to work are understandably anxious about making sure their baby will take a bottle, but try not to let the short time you have together be spoilt by fretting about this.

Q What if she won't take a bottle?

A A baby who enjoys breastfeeding may not particularly welcome having milk from a bottle, especially when her mother is available. The first strategy could be to get other people to try – your partner or your childminder for example – while you keep out of sight. She may be happy doing things for other people that she won't do with you. You could also try holding your baby in a different position from your usual breastfeeding one – facing outwards for instance. Experiment with temperatures – some babies will drink milk from a bottle at body temperature, like breastmilk, while others prefer it cool or at room temperature. You can try a variety of bottle teats, and have a go at softening them with warm, boiled water. If your baby really won't accept a bottle, then it is possible to feed her with a spoon or a soft-spouted beaker. If she's around six months, she might manage to drink from a beaker. Some babies never bottle-feed, moving happily from breastfeeding to using a cup as part of the family meal. You can continue to breastfeed when you go back to work, feeding at nights, early in the morning and at weekends. If your working days are relatively short, your baby might decide to wait until you come home and then enjoy a very long feed.

I went back to work part-time when Robert was nine months old. During the day, the childminder gave him food and water from a cup and then we used to have a breastfeed as soon as I got back from work. For both of us, it was a lovely way of re-connecting after a tiring day.

Emma

Myth or Fact?

While you are Breastfeeding, your Vagina may be drier than normal

Fact. Any dryness is hormonal, and not an indication of 'frigidity'. You can resume sex whenever you feel like it, but you may need to use a lubricant gel.

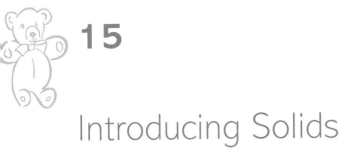

15

Introducing Solids

Introducing solids should be a gradual process, and your baby's first solid foods are simply for practice. He needs lots of energy for growing which he can't get from solids alone, so milk will remain his primary source of nutrients until he is at least 12 months old.

In the past, many babies were started on solid foods too early. Research shows that babies' digestive systems are not adapted to digest foods other than milk before about six months of age. So breastmilk is all most babies need for about the first six months. If they are given solid foods earlier, they just take less breastmilk. They are also more likely to develop eczema, respiratory diseases and become overweight if started on solid foods before about four months.

For formula-fed babies, there is less research evidence, but good reasons not to start solids before 17 weeks. However, it is important to tune in to your baby's own cues that he is ready to start.

Ask yourself whether your baby is ready for solids. Does he:

- pick up small things and put them in his mouth
- sit up and hold his head up firmly
- watch you eat with great interest
- seem hungry again soon after a feed?

If you think your baby is really ready to try solid foods, then you can try offering him a teaspoon or so, after a breastfeed. Good early foods to try are puréed vegetables or fruit, and non-gluten cereals, such as ground or baby rice mixed with expressed breastmilk or water, without any additional sugar or salt. If you have a family history of allergies, it's best to introduce new foods one at a time, a few days apart. That way, if your baby reacts to any substance, you will be able to identify it quite easily.

Your Baby's Diet

Over the next few years your baby will establish eating habits, which have long-term implications for his health. If you have never really thought about what you eat before, this may be a good time to turn over a new leaf for your baby's sake.

- *Carbohydrates* – rice, pasta, bread, potatoes. These should form the bulk of your family's diet. Whole-grain cereals contain more essential nutrients as they have undergone less processing. However, your baby cannot cope with too much fibre, so a mixture of whole-grain cereals with some refined products may be a good idea. Once your baby is eating with you, loose stools are a sign that he may have too much fibre in his diet.

If your family has a history of coeliac disease, you are recommended to leave wheat-based products like pasta and bread out of your baby's diet for at least a year.

- *Protein* – meat, fish, cheese, nuts, legumes. We all need some protein in our diets, but most of us consume too much. Protein foods tend to be good sources of vitamins and minerals.

- *Fats* – Although adults should aim for a low-fat diet, babies and toddlers obtain much of their energy from fat, so need higher proportions of healthy fats. Your baby needs roughly half the energy or calories you do, but as his stomach is so much smaller, he cannot cope with large quantities of foods. Avoid cow's milk for general drinking under 12 months, but after that use full-fat milk until he is at least two years old. Soya milks and milks from other animals such as goats and sheep are best avoided at this stage.

Families with a history of eczema and asthma are recommended to introduce dairy products slowly, ideally avoiding them in the first year.

- *Fruit and vegetables* should be another essential part of our diet, not only as a source of vitamins, but also for fibre. Raw fruit and vegetables are particularly healthy. Try to vary the groups your family eats – greens (spinach, lettuce, peas) and oranges (apricots, carrots, orange peppers) will provide different nutrients. Buy fruit and vegetables as fresh as you can, store them in the fridge until you need them and cook quickly – steaming or microwaving preserves more vitamins. Dried and fresh fruits can be given as healthy between-meal snacks.

Most fruits and vegetables are easily tolerated, although children under one year often have difficulty with citrus fruits (like oranges) and occasionally with strawberries.

- *Calcium* – essential for your baby's growing bones, it comes from not only milk, cheese and yoghurt but also from sources such as dark green vegetables and ground sesame seeds (tahini paste).

Hot and spicy and salty foods are too difficult for your baby to digest. Nuts are a choking hazard, and peanuts can trigger allergies – so avoid these products until he is much older.

Babies are programmed to like sweet things, because breastmilk is sweet. However, the sweetness of breastmilk is due to lactose, which is much less likely to cause tooth decay than refined sugar. Your child will get plenty of natural sugars such as fructose in fruit and lactose in milk, so there is no need to add any more to their food. Artificial sweeteners are unsuitable for children under three.

Convenience Foods

Jars and packets of commercial baby foods can be convenient when you're out and about. However, processed baby foods have some drawbacks, so use them sparingly, and always check that they are suitable for your baby's age.

- Initially, there will be waste, as your baby will only eat a couple of teaspoonfuls per meal.
- They don't always taste like 'real food', and if you use them a lot your baby may reject your own cooking.
- They are more expensive than home cooking.
- It can be hard to judge allergic reactions as some jars contain several different ingredients – read the labels carefully to avoid such things as dairy products if that is important to you.

Home-made 'Convenience' Foods

- Mashed organic banana or avocado – convenient instant foods when travelling.
- Remove the skin of a mango with a sharp knife. Roughly chop the flesh off the stone, liquidize and serve.
- Steam a cube of frozen spinach until defrosted and evenly heated, then mix with baby rice and milk.

To purée vegetables:

- Either boil in small amount of water, or steam (perhaps above your own meal) until soft.
- Liquidize using the cooking water if boiled, adding more water as necessary until the mixture is very smooth and just runny enough to plop off a spoon.
- Excess mixture can be frozen in ice cube trays, and defrosted as needed.

Your Questions Answered

Q **My breastfed baby is completely uninterested in solid foods. Is there anything I can do?**

A If he is under six months, you could try again in a couple of weeks or so. Is he offered solids after a breastfeed? He might be full. Try sitting him at the family table, and if he looks interested, offer him a portion. Babies love to copy. Perhaps he would prefer to feed himself? Could you try finger food such as squashy sandwiches? Try to be relaxed yourself about it; as long as he's thriving there's probably no need to worry. If you're not sure, then ask your GP to check his overall development.

Q **My breastfed baby put on lots of weight early on, but now he is 12 weeks old, he is not keeping up with his line on the growth chart. Should I put him on solids?**

A Many of the growth charts now in use were drawn up when the majority of babies were being bottle-fed, although there were new charts drawn up in 2001 for breastfed babies – ask your health visitor which one you have. It seems that breastfed babies gain weight faster initially, but this starts to slow, showing a levelling-off according to the charts at about this age. As long as your baby isn't losing weight, but is still growing, even if not as quickly as before, and is alert, there is unlikely to be cause for concern. The most important indicators of growth are length and head circumference, not weight. In any case, you should not introduce solids too soon, as your baby's gut is too immature to cope with them, and early solids can cause health problems later in life. If your baby is less than six months and seems to need more food, you can try increasing the amount of milk you give him at feeds, or offer more frequent feeds.

Q **When exactly is the recommended age for introducing solids?**

A Views have changed about when babies should be starting solid foods. Following recent research, UNICEF and the World Health Organization now recommend that babies receive only breast-milk until they are at least six months old. In Britain, these guidelines have not yet been adopted, so health professionals still recommend introducing solids between four and six months.

Myth or Fact?

Breastfeeding can Help you Lose Weight

Fact. During pregnancy, your body lays down extra stores of fat in preparation for breastfeeding. Although some women lose the extra weight easily while breastfeeding, others find their weight doesn't reduce until they stop. If you eat nutritious foods to satisfy your appetite and no more, you should lose weight more easily by breast-feeding, whereas if you bottle-feed, you will have to make an effort to lose this weight.

16

When to Stop Breastfeeding

You are breastfeeding, and everything seems to be going well. So when should you stop? And who should make that decision – you, your baby or the rest of your family?

Even though breastfeeding is far more socially acceptable in this country than it was even a few years ago, most mothers in the UK will not breastfeed their babies for long. Many women give up because of returning to work, while others stop in the early weeks because they find breastfeeding difficult. Some mothers, despite enjoying breast-feeding, are pressurized into stopping before they really feel ready to do so.

There is no right or wrong time to stop – the decision is entirely personal, and will depend on you, your baby and your own unique cir-cumstances. Whatever you decide, breastfeeding for any length of time – be it three or four days or three or four years – will give your child a head start and is well worth doing.

Reasons Women Consider Weaning

The Grizzly Baby

Because weaning is something you can control, it can be tempting to stop breastfeeding when you are trying to solve another problem – maybe your baby is clingy or grizzly. Unfortunately, what can happen then is that the problem doesn't go away, but you lose one of your comforters! If now doesn't feel like the right time to wean, look for other solutions first. It may just be that your child is going through a grizzly patch (*see Chapter* 9).

The Baby who Wakes a Lot at Night

Far more children wake during the night than most parenting books would have us believe. It is unlikely that your baby wakes up because she's breastfed. If you change to formula feeding, your sleep will still be disturbed by having to heat up bottles. If your baby is a few months old, and still waking more than once a night, it is worth talking this over with a breastfeeding counsellor or health visitor, as they may be able to suggest changes to your night-time routines (*see Chapter* 8).

Starting Solids

Introducing solids doesn't mean you need to wean your baby from your breast. It's a good idea to keep breastfeeds going, in fact, as then you can be sure your baby is getting a good, balanced diet. Your baby will still need breastmilk or formula milk as her main form of nutrition until she is at least 12 months old (*see the previous chapter*).

Returning to Work

This is a time when many mothers feel they 'ought' to wean their baby, but in fact there is no need to do so, even if returning full time. Keeping breastfeeds going can feel very important – an intimate way of linking up with your baby after being apart all day (*see Chapter* 14).

Deciding to Continue

If your baby wants to continue feeding after her peers have stopped, this does not say anything in particular about her. It doesn't mean she's too clingy, or that he will grow up to be a mummy's boy. If anything, children who feel very secure early in life often grow up to be more outgoing and independent, whereas the child who was forced into independence too early can often remain anxious and insecure for a long time.

It can be hard, however, to continue breastfeeding when your relatives disapprove. Talking it through does sometimes help. Your mother gave birth to you at a time when breastfeeding was made very difficult, and may feel a sense of failure at her own very different experience – or may feel your feeding choice is an implied criticism of hers.

If you are under pressure to give up breastfeeding before you and your baby really want to, it may be helpful to remember that the majority of babies in the world are nursed well into their second year, and in many societies toddlers are still breastfed when they are three, four or even five years old. Not so long ago, in our culture too, children were nursed far longer than they are now.

You will need to think about what you and your baby are going to call breastfeeds, before she starts talking. Some mothers are embarrassed into stopping when their child starts demanding 'boobies', so choose a word that you don't mind – a baby word like 'milks' or a euphemism like 'cuddles' can work well.

Weaning when you Want to, but your Baby Doesn't

As with all changes, try to avoid a time in your baby's life when other, stressful things are going on. For example, weaning just before returning to work, going on holiday or when potty training is likely to be more difficult. During the summer is a good time if you are both going out a lot and doing interesting things – it is easier to distract her. Times when you are stuck indoors are hard – a seated mother is a real temptation for a breastfed child.

To cut out a bedtime feed, choose a week when other people can put her to bed, and think of some other methods of comfort – reading stories, lots of soft toys to cuddle up to, lullaby tapes playing softly. You will need to be prepared for some tears, and you should think through beforehand how far you are prepared to go. If your child is utterly distraught and won't be comforted, don't feel you are 'failing' if you decide to back down for the moment. She may well find it far easier in a few months' time.

Weaning by Mutual Consent

Breastfeeding has nutritional and emotional benefits for as long as you both choose to do it. If you leave nature to take its course, weaning will happen gradually. Breastfeeding will become less important for your child, something to lay aside as she becomes more independent.

Weaning will become easier as she develops outside interests and becomes less focused on you. In the end, all she may need is just a bit of positive encouragement from you to give up this baby attachment, in the same way as you will encourage her to take her first steps, to use the toilet and other milestones on the road to independence.

Top Weaning Tips

- Cut down on breastfeeds gradually – otherwise you will get engorged, and may get mastitis.
- Cut out one feed at a time – express just enough to make yourself comfortable.
- Leave a few days – up to a week if possible – before cutting out the next feed.

Re-starting

If you wean your baby and then regret it, you may be able to start again or 're-lactate'. A breastfeeding counsellor can offer help and support. It will be far easier to do if:

- it is not very long since you stopped
- breastfeeding was well established before
- you have access to a battery or electric pump.

Grandmothers in other cultures sometimes re-lactate in order to feed orphaned grandchildren – even after menopause. So anything is possible!

Your Questions Answered

Q Do I need to stop breastfeeding if I want to get pregnant?

A A few women will not ovulate until they have stopped breastfeeding completely, so if you are finding it hard to conceive, this may be the reason. More often than not, however, you will start to ovulate while you are still nursing. If you become pregnant while you are still breastfeeding your older child, you can continue to feed your baby (*for more details, see* Appendix 1).

Q How do I stop breastfeeding quickly? I need to go into hospital.

A Stopping breastfeeding suddenly can cause problems, but sometimes it's unavoidable. Try talking through your options with someone to see if there are any alternatives – most hospitals will let mothers bring breastfed babies in with them, for example. But if it's really necessary, then:

- express only a little milk to relieve the pressure inside your breasts – no more
- wear a firm, comfortable bra
- you may need something like paracetamol if the pressure feels painful
- if the pressure buildup gets bad, especially if you start to feel unwell, then use an electric pump to empty your breasts entirely *on one occasion only*. From then on, go back to taking off small amounts when the pressure gets too much.

You could consider re-lactating when you get out of hospital.

Myth or Fact?

Breastfeeding Drains you – Bottle-feeding is Less Tiring

Myth. Breastfeeding doesn't 'drain' you; but being a new mother is very tiring. It will take quite a while to recover physically from the birth, and to get used to looking after a tiny baby. Try to keep other demands to a minimum, and ask for help and support.

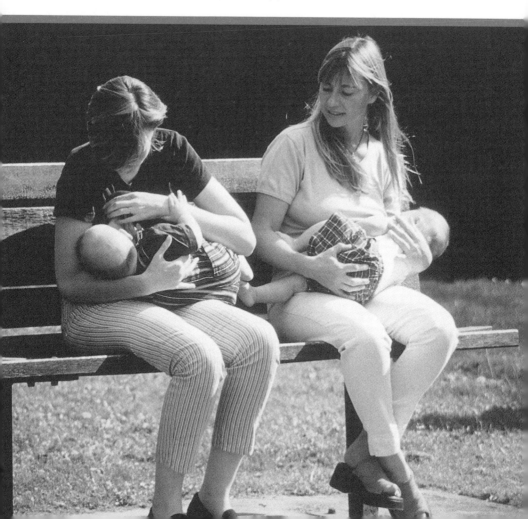

Questions and Answers

Q
Will breastfeeding work as a form of birth control?

A
Breastfeeding is an effective method of birth control, but only if certain conditions are met, and like all contraception, it is not foolproof. Breastfeeding delays the return of your periods. However, the first time you ovulate after giving birth will be *before* your first period, and you have a 10 per cent risk of falling pregnant if you rely solely on your period returning as a warning that you are fertile. Scientists have defined LAM (Lactational Amenorrhoea Method – relying on absence of periods while breastfeeding) as 98–99 per cent effective only if:

- you are breastfeeding your baby on demand, night and day, without using any supplements (usually meaning at least ten short or six long breastfeeds within 24 hours with no interval between feeds of more than six hours and no use of dummies)
- your baby is less than six months old.

Once this changes – such as when you introduce solids – LAM can continue to be effective if your periods still haven't returned as long as you are taught to keep an eye out for ovulation occurring using other natural fertility control methods. These include observation of cervical mucus or recording basal body temperature. The risk of falling pregnant using LAM plus these observational methods is less than 2 per cent again, even for a breastfed baby of over six months.

If it is vital that you do not conceive again, you might want to use additional precautions such as condoms. Check that a diaphragm continues to fit well if you are losing weight. We don't know if there are any long-term effects on babies, particularly boys, of exposure to female hormones in the contraceptive pill. Oestrogen suppresses lactation, and so the combined pill would reduce your milk supply; therefore the progesterone only (mini) pill is usually offered to breastfeeding mothers, although this also briefly reduces supply.

Q Can I breastfeed with pierced nipples?

A Many women with pierced nipples go on to breastfeed their babies successfully, although there is anecdotal evidence that horizontal piercing is better suited to breastfeeding. There have been incidences of women breastfeeding without removing their nipple rings, but most health professionals agree that breastfeeding with nipple jewellery does cause problems for the baby, which are solved when jewellery is removed. It may also be dangerous for your baby to feed while jewellery is in place, in case it becomes dislodged and chokes him. In addition, his gums, tongue or palate could be damaged by nipple jewellery.

It's possible to have the rings removed, and then replaced when you stop breastfeeding, if the piercing took place a while ago. The average healing time for nipples is three to six months, though many piercers believe it takes longer. Contact a piercer for assistance in taking them out.

Q Is it possible to continue breastfeeding my son whilst pregnant with my next baby?

A Yes – your body will carry on producing milk throughout your pregnancy. It's even possible to continue feeding your son after your new baby is born – this is called 'tandem feeding'.

Breastfeeding during pregnancy is fine for most women, although it's important to eat well. Hormonal changes in the early days may give you sensitive nipples, making breastfeeding difficult. Nipple stimulation, through breastfeeding or making love, will cause mild uterine contractions, but for most women these are not strong enough to create a problem. However, if you have a history of premature delivery or miscarriage, or if you are bleeding, then you might need to think about weaning your older child, although opinions do differ on this.

During the fourth or fifth month of your pregnancy, your milk reverts to colostrum, so taste changes and volume decreases. Some children decide to wean themselves at this point, although others persevere. If your child wants to continue, don't worry about using your colostrum up; your body will continue to produce this special milk until your new baby needs it. If your child is under a year old and therefore nutritionally dependent on your milk, you might need to keep track of his weight gain at this point.

It is worth thinking about whether you want to continue feeding an older child once your new baby arrives. If tandem feeding is not for you, then it'll probably be less traumatic for your older child to wean in pregnancy rather than waiting until the new baby arrives when he is in danger of feeling usurped anyway. If you are not yet pregnant, but trying, it can be harder to conceive while still breastfeeding, as some women find they don't ovulate until they wean.

It is perfectly possible to breastfeed an older child and new baby together, but you will need to be extra careful to get a good diet and plenty of rest; it's like breastfeeding twins. You will also need to make sure that the new baby has enough to eat, so usually he will need to go the breast first. However, your older child will help keep your milk supply going, which can be useful if your newborn is slow to start breastfeeding.

Can I breastfeed ...

With inverted or flat nipples?

Yes, these are quite normal and often the baby will draw them out when he feeds. The problem can be getting positioning just right. You will need to line him up 'nose to nipple' so that when baby opens his mouth wide and you move him onto your breast, your nipple will contact the roof of his mouth. If you squeeze your areola between your fingers, you should feel a harder centre; this is your nipple stem; use this as your guide.

After surgery to correct an inverted nipple?

Unfortunately, you may have had the milk ducts severed. Talk to your surgeon to see if this was the case. Some breastfeeding may still be possible as ducts can re-grow to some extent.

After breast reduction?

Yes, breastfeeding should be possible. Ask your surgeon whether milk ducts were severed, but you probably won't know until you try.

After treatment for cancer?

If you had radiation or a mastectomy, you probably won't be able to feed on the affected side, but the other breast will still work fine. You will need to put your baby to your unaffected breast as often as possible in the early days to make sure it produces enough milk on its own. After a lumpectomy, breastfeeding should be possible on both sides.

With implants?
Implants don't affect breastfeeding. The silicone should not affect the baby – formula milk has even been found to have higher silicone levels than women's breastmilk, with or without implants.

Q I think I have too much milk! I am always leaking, and when my baby goes on, he seems to choke a bit at first. Now he often fights me, and this is quite distressing. What can I do?

A A few women do in fact produce more milk than their baby wants, and this can be distressing. You could try expressing off a little milk at the beginning of a feed, just to avoid that first rush. Then if you sit your baby as upright as possible, this should help him. Some mothers occasionally even feed lying down with their baby on top of them!

If he comes off quickly because of your flow, put him back to the same side, otherwise you may over-stimulate your breasts, producing too much milk by swapping sides too often. The more your baby stimulates your breasts, the more milk you produce, and if you have a huge supply, it will mean that he has more foremilk to drink before the hindmilk comes through. Ironically, many mothers start to believe that they don't have enough milk if their baby wants to feed all the time when in fact they have a copious supply.

Most women find that this oversupply will ease by six or eight weeks. You can press on the other breast with the heel of your hand to try to stop the leakage. Wearing dark, loose, patterned tops will disguise leaks. Some women who suffer a lot from leaking find it helps to splash cold water on their nipples.

Q Why are my baby's stools often green?

A baby who is being exclusively breastfed usually has stools which are bright yellow, sweet smelling and the consistency of scrambled eggs. If you introduce anything else into a baby's diet, like formula or solids, then the stools will change, usually to become more like an adult's – more brown, solid and foul-smelling.

Green stools in a baby who is receiving nothing but breast-milk are a warning sign that there is an imbalance. If your baby's stools are nearly always green and if he is not gaining weight well, even though your milk supply seems fine, then it could be that he is getting too much fore milk and not enough hind milk. As the fore milk is more dilute, with more lactose and fewer calories, it stimulates your baby's digestive tract to move the milk along too fast, producing green, often explosive, nappies! You can try waiting until your baby finishes the first breast, and so gets enough hind milk, before offering the second breast; it may even be that he will only need one breast per feed. You could also ask a breastfeeding counsellor to check that your baby's positioning and attachment is good enough for him to extract all the rich hind milk.

Consistently green stools could also, however, be a warning that your baby is sensitive to something. Is he on any medication? If not, could he be sensitive to medications you are taking, like iron supplements? Very occasionally, a baby can become sensitive to something in his mother's diet which is passed to him through her breastmilk. Often other symptoms are present, like eczema or a rash. It can be hard to pinpoint the trigger, so if you suspect your baby has a food intolerance, you could talk it through with a dietician or breastfeeding counsellor.

Contacts

National Childbirth Trust
See page 131.

Ameda Egnell Ltd
Breast pumps to hire or buy. Unit 1, Belvedere Trading Estate, Taunton, Somerset TA1 1BH. Tel: 01823 336362.

BLISS
Information for parents of premature babies. 2nd Floor, Albert Embankment, London SE1 7OP. Tel: 0207 820 471. You can also call their free helpline on 0500 618 140, visit their website: www.bliss.org.uk or e-mail them at information@bliss.org.uk

The Maternity Alliance
For information and advice on employment rights and help with negotiating conditions while breastfeeding. 45 Beech Street, London EC2P 2LX. Tel: 0207 588 8582.

Medela
Breast pumps to hire or buy; also sells purified lanolin as a nipple cream. Tel: 01538 386650.

Parents at work

Support and information for working mothers. 45 Beech Street, London EC2Y 8AD. Tel: 0207 628 3578.

Serene

For help with babies who cry a lot. Tel: 0207 404 5011, 9am till 11pm.

TAMBA (Twins And Multiple Births Association)

Leaflets and booklets on all aspects of looking after twins or more. Harnott House, 309 Chester Road, Little Sutton, Ellesmere Port CH66 1QQ. Tel: 0151 348 0020. They can put you in touch with your local **twins club,** and run **Twinline**, confidential listening service 7–11pm weekdays, 10am-11pm weekends. Tel: 01732 868000.

UNICEF UK Baby Friendly Initiative

A global campaign to support every mother's right to choose breastfeeding for her baby, funded by the United Nations Children's Fund (UNICEF). Africa House, 64–78 Kingsway, London WC2B 6NB. Tel: 0207 312 7652, www.babyfriendly.org.uk

YMCA England

For postnatal exercise. The YMCA runs fitness classes in centres all over the UK. To find your local centre, write to 3–9 Southampton Row, London WC1B 5HY or phone 0208 520 5599, e-mail: enquiries@ymca.org.uk or visit their website: www.ymca.org.uk

Ten Steps to Successful Breastfeeding

The 'Ten Steps to Successful Breastfeeding' are the foundation of the Baby Friendly Hospital Initiative (BFHI), set up by the World Health Organization (WHO) and the United Nations Children's Fund (UNICEF). They sum up the maternity practices necessary to support breastfeeding.

Every facility providing maternity services and care for newborn infants should:

1 Have a written breastfeeding policy that is routinely communicated to all health care staff.

2 Train all health care staff in skills necessary to implement this policy.

3 Inform all pregnant women about the benefits and management of breastfeeding.

4 Help mothers initiate breastfeeding soon after birth.

5 Show mothers how to breastfeed and how to maintain lactation even if they should be separated from their infants.

6 Give newborn infants no food or drink other than breastmilk, unless medically indicated.

7 Practise rooming-in – allowing mothers and infants to remain together – 24 hours a day.

8 Encourage breastfeeding on demand.

9 Give no artificial teats or pacifiers (also called dummies or soothers) to breastfeeding infants.

10 Foster the establishment of breastfeeding support groups and refer mothers to them on discharge from the hospital or clinic.

About the
National Childbirth Trust

Run by parents, for parents, the National Childbirth Trust is a self-help charity organization with 400 branches across the UK. There's bound to be a local branch near you, running:

- childbirth classes
- breastfeeding counselling
- new baby groups
- open house get-togethers
- support for dads
- working-parents' groups
- nearly-new sales of baby clothes and equipment

– as well as loads of events where you can meet and make friends with other people going through the same changes.

- To find the contact details of your local branch, ring the NCT Enquiries Line: 0870 444 8707.
- To get support with feeding your baby, ring the NCT Breastfeeding Line: 0870 444 8708. Any day, 8am to 10pm.
- To find answers to pregnancy queries, ring the Enquiries Line or log on to: www.nctpregnancyandbabycare.com

- To buy excellent baby goods, maternity bras, toys and gifts, call 0141 636 0600 or look at: www.nctms.co.uk
- To join the NCT, just call 0870 990 8040 with a credit card.

You don't have to become a member to enjoy the services and support of the National Childbirth Trust. It's open to everyone. We do encourage people to join the charity because it helps fund our work – supporting all parents.

When you become an NCT member and join your local group, you'll get a regular neighbourhood newsletter (a guide to your area aimed at new parents) and you'll also receive NCT's *New Generation* – our mailed-out members' magazine that takes an in-depth look at all issues of interest to new parents.

'The NCT support network is second to none. It's very reassuring and comforting.'

The National Childbirth Trust wants all parents to have an experience of pregnancy, birth and early parenthood that enriches their lives and gives them confidence in being a parent.

National Childbirth Trust
Alexandra House
Oldham Terrace
London W3 6NH
Tel: 0870 770 3236
Fax: 0870 770 3237

Index